Syndrome

A Comprehensive Guide For
Understanding, Living With, And
Treating Asperger Syndrome

By Frank Ryan

Table of Contents

Introduction

I want to thank and congratulate you for deciding to read this book entitled, *Asperger Syndrome: A Comprehensive Guide for Understanding, Living with and Treating Asperger Syndrome.*

Many people now know about autism and autistics. For some patients and a few outside observers, one of the worst things about autism is the pity people feel for and treat patients of autism with. In 2013, autism was classified as a spectrum of various disorders, one of which is the Asperger Syndrome, also known as Asperger's Syndrome, Asperger Disorder or simply, Asperger's. The patients of the disorder refer to themselves as *aspies*.

In an uncharacteristic naming process, the disorder was not named after the person who discovered it. It was named after pediatrician *Hans Asperger* from Austria, who exhibited the symptoms of the syndrome as a child. After he became a pediatrician, Asperger reported some children in his care as patients of "autistic psychopathy," as he called it. It wasn't until 50 years later that the disorder was identified as a separate medical condition.

Autism and Asperger Syndrome belong to a group of *neurodevelopmental disorders.* The term describes impairments in the development and growth of the brain or the central nervous system that result from the existence of multiple issues and mechanisms, the most important of which is genetic contribution, even though no specific gene has yet been identified.

The syndrome is accompanied by significant problems with social interaction, nonverbal communication and behavioral and interest patterns. The underlying causes seem to affect many or all functional brain systems, instead of being localized. Unfortunately, science and research have not yet identified the specific underpinnings of the disorder.

The relevant neuroanatomical studies seem to point to the direction of alteration of the brain development soon after the embryo has been conceived, due to abnormal migration of embryonic cells during the development of the fetus. The end result of these abnormal migrations is the alteration of the neural circuits that are responsible for controlling the thought and behavioral processes.

Asperger's is so new that no reliable tools for the diagnosis have been developed yet. Initially, it generally depends on the parents, to notice the differences in the development of their own child, and on a general practitioner or a pediatrician, to identify the signs and further investigate the problem. There are several screening instruments that can be used, but a second opinion would always be necessary as the diagnosis is very difficult and may not differentiate from other disorders on the autism spectrum.

Once it has been diagnosed and the diagnosis has been confirmed, the syndrome is managed through medication and teaching. And here lies another problem as no Asperger Syndrome specific medication has been developed and, actually, the patients are often used for experimentation. The atypical antipsychotics *risperidone* and *olanzapine* seem to show more promise than the selective serotonin reuptake inhibitors (SSRIs), which have also been tested.

It is more likely for better results to be achieved through *teaching* the patients the skills of social interaction, communication and vocation that they did not acquire through their normal development. The intervention must be tailor made for each specific individual, and it must be based on a multidisciplinary assessment of the patient. It is unfortunate that all pertinent information regarding the effectiveness of the teaching is not yet enough to produce a reasonably sound outcome.

Modern medicine considers the syndrome as a disorder that needs a cure. But a recent issue says that the patients themselves do not consider Asperger's as a disorder or as anything that needs treatment. They consider themselves as simply being different from the rest of the world, as they consider that there is no ideal brain configuration. Based on this notion, they raise the point that people who are diagnosed with the syndrome are not treated unless the patient requests treatment.

Through their subculture called *Wrong Planet*, they advocate that the syndrome is neither a disorder nor a disability, that it should be treated the same as homosexuality, and that it should be removed from the Diagnostic and Statistical Manual. Simon Baron-Cohen even went so far as to write that some of the characteristics displayed by aspies are to be cherished and not considered shortcomings. According to him, the only reasons to still consider aspies as patients is to ensure that they receive the legally required special support and to identify possible emotional difficulties.

The issue should further be limited only to adults who still display the effects of the syndrome after they have reached adulthood. This is because these symptoms are gradually reduced as the aspie grows up. Approximately 20% of people diagnosed with the syndrome as children do not display any symptoms of Asperger's after reaching adulthood. But since the disorder begins its course in childhood, it would be rather difficult, if not impossible, to persuade parents to let their children remain this way and not to seek treatment.

As the title suggests, the first step is to understand the condition. Fortunately, people no longer consider what they do not understand as some form of witchcraft. This provides the aspie with the chance to identify the condition, seek professional guidance and live a normal life, once the appropriate measures are implemented.

At this point, it should be stated that the contents of this book in no way attempt to replace or override the suggested treatment of an appropriately trained professional. On the contrary, it is strongly recommended that such advice and guidance is sought before any decisions as to the treatment of an aspie are taken. Medical professionals are the only ones properly qualified to provide such services.

One final reason to ask for professional advice is that apart from the mainstream options for medication, there are also alternative natural treatments that may be used. Should the choice be made to divert from mainstream medicine and try any of the alternative treatments, there could be a number of side effects involved that patients should be aware of.

Whether you consider Asperger's a disorder or not, living a normal life under this condition is absolutely feasible and achievable. The following chapters will show you how.

Thanks again for deciding to read this book, I hope you enjoy it!

Chapter 1: Overview of the Asperger Syndrome

It is unfortunate that children sometimes show signs and symptoms which have been attributed to neurodevelopmental disorders. These disorders have to do with social deficits, difficulties in communication, repetitive behaviors, intensely focused interests, issues in sensory perception, and sometimes delays in cognitive functions.

Before 2013, all of the above were classified as **autism**. After careful studies, it was discovered that four different and distinct disorders existed, and therefore, what was previously known and defined as *autism*, would hence forth be named **autism spectrum** or **autistic spectrum of disorders**. The differences lie mostly in the symptoms exhibited in each case. The four distinct disorders are:

A) Pervasive developmental disorder not otherwise specified (PDD-NOS).
    The condition is diagnosed whenever the symptoms exhibited do not match the

criteria defined in any of the other three categories. This classification is also one of the five pervasive developmental disorders that are not necessarily associated with any form of autism.

To receive a diagnosis, it is necessary for a team of specialists to be involved in the process and that an individual suspected of displaying PDD-NOS undergoes a full set of diagnostic evaluations, including:

➢ Thorough examination of the historical record in social, adaptive, and motor skills, as well as communication and medical issues.
➢ Scores on behavioral rating scales.
➢ Observations of current behavioral patterns.
➢ Psychological evaluation.
➢ Educational evaluation.
➢ Evaluation of the current communication skills.
➢ Evaluating of the current occupation.

Researchers face a methodology problem with PDD-NOS, as the group of people who are diagnosed is heterogeneous and there is but only a brief case definition of PDD-NOS as a "sub-threshold" category.

It would appear from the clinical evidence that there are fewer intellectual deficits involved for children with PDD-NOS than in classical autism. Additionally, it is possible for these children to be submitted for evaluation at a later age than with the other three disorders of the autism spectrum.

B) Childhood disintegrative disorder

The condition is also known as the ***Heller's Syndrome*** or ***disintegrative psychosis***. The characteristics defining this disorder are delays in the development of age-relevant language, poor social interactions and weak motor skills. This was actually the first form of autism to be discovered in 1908, and it is also the rarest. Theodor Heller, who initially described it (and consequently gave his name), called it *dementia infantilis*.

Perhaps the most crucial characteristic of this condition is that it is not made apparent immediately. In the majority of cases, there is a period of normal development for the child before the problems begin to appear. In some cases, this regression is so dramatic that the child is not even aware of it and will never ask about what is happening to him or her.

Most of the time, it is diagnosed when previously attained skills have been lost. It can happen any time during the normal development of a child, but typically onset is around the age of three. The skills that may be lost are included in at least two of the following six areas of developmental functionalities:

- The ability to produce speech coherent enough to communicate a message. This is also known as *expressive language*.
- The ability to listen to others and understand the message that is communicated. Also known as *receptive language*.
- Skills that pertain to social and self-care issues.
- Control of the bladder and bowel movements.
- The ability of imaginative play.
- Motor skills.

For these six classifications, the once-acquired skills have been almost completely lost between the ages of 2 and 10. But in order for the diagnosis to be CDD, there must also be impairment or complete absence in at least two of the following areas:

➢ Social interaction
➢ Communication
➢ Patterns of restrictive and repetitive behavior and / or interests

CDD is also a disorder classification of which some of the underlying causes have been identified. (It has been linked with lipid storage diseases, subacute sclerosing panencephalitis and tuberous sclerosis.) These findings have raised considerable debates and controversies in reference to the right methods of treatment.

C) Classical Autism

If a child begins to display, within the first years of his or her life, symptoms of impaired social interaction, difficulties in verbal and non-verbal communication and behavioral patterns that are restricted and repetitive, it is most probable that the diagnosis will be standard autism.

This disorder is attributed to genetic and environmental issues, along with the use of agents that may cause birth defects. It is highly heritable, and for a successful diagnosis, the prerequisite is that the symptoms appear before the age of three.

Unlike with Asperger Syndrome, after the onset of autism there are only a small number of patients that can take care of themselves without supervision once they have reached adulthood.

A worrisome statistic is that the percentage of the appearance of autism within the general population has increased dramatically since the 1980s and the standardization of diagnostic tests. As of 2010, it was estimated that 1 or 2 individuals out of every 1,000 people on a worldwide basis suffer from classical autism. While it is not sex discriminant, the frequency of onset is five times greater in boys than in girls.

D) Asperger Syndrome
The condition is characterized by the presence of all the symptoms that appear in the autism spectrum of disorders:

- ➢ Difficulty in social functionality and interaction
- ➢ Difficulty in verbal and non-verbal communication
- ➢ Patterns of restricted and repetitive behavior
- ➢ Restrictive and repetitive interests
- ➢ Physical clumsiness
- ➢ Atypical use of language

The last two symptoms are not required for the diagnosis of the syndrome, but they are present very frequently among the patients.

The discussion in this book will focus on Asperger Syndrome, its characteristics, classification, and all of the pertinent details which will allow for a better understanding. In addition, the accumulation of knowledge about the circumstances and reference information will help clarify what it is and what can be done about it.

Causes

Science and research have not yet defined what exactly it is that causes the syndrome. Part of the hypothesis formed thus far includes genetic factors, but a certain genetic cause or gene has yet to be identified. Nor was brain imaging successful in defining a common pathology, and there is only very limited and sketchy information on the effects of particular interventions.

Furthermore, there is no single treatment that can address all the symptoms and work on all patients. Currently the sets of remedies explored have focused on behavioral therapy that addresses the specific inadequacies and deficits presented on a case-by-case basis.

Returning to the genetic hypothesis of Asperger's, this is supported by the observations of a phenotypic variability that has been seen in children suffering from AS. For the uninitiated, phenotypes are the composites of an organism's traits or observable characteristics. These include morphology, biochemical properties, physiological properties, as well as the organism's behavior and its products (the nest of a bird is a product of the bird's behavior, for example).

Further evidence is provided by the fact that the syndrome tends to run in families and that the genetic component in this syndrome appears to be stronger than the genetic component found in the other disorders of the autistic spectrum.

It is also possible that siblings may display similar symptoms but at different intensities and that one member of the family may actually be diagnosable with AS, while the other members exhibit similar behaviors but in a much more limited form which is not actually diagnosable.

There is a working hypothesis undergoing research that involves a common group of genes where the presence of some particular *alleles* may result in a greater vulnerability of an individual developing AS. Should this indeed be the case, it is the combination of the alleles involved that determines the severity of the disorder and the intensity of the symptoms exhibited.

For those not familiar with the biology, an *allele* is something like an isotope. Genes are not always exactly the same. They appear in a number of alternative forms. One of these alternative forms is called an allele. The best example of what an allele is may be the color of the skin. The difference between Asian, Caucasian, and African races in terms of the color of the skin is based on a different allele of the same gene.

The same stands true if the allele does not refer to a specific gene but a *gene locus,* which is actually the location within a gene, a chromosome or a DNA sequence in which an allele is found. It may even be that a specific DNA sequence that is found in a specific location is, itself, an allele.

For those who want to study the allele hypothesis further, they should first acquire further knowledge of the human genome and the genetic maps, as these are where determining the location of a specific biological trait is occurring.

Further scientific observations link Asperger's to exposure of the mother to teratogen agents within the first eight weeks of conception. Teratogens are the agents that cause birth defects. Some teratogens are:

A) *Toxic substances* such as drugs
   Either for pharmaceutical or for recreational purposes, any medical compounds that act during the embryonic and fetal development may produce an alteration in a form or a function.

B) Environmental toxins

There is evidence that:

> Polychlorinated biphenyls
> Phthalates
> Phenols
> Organo-chlorine pesticides
> Polybrominated diphenyl ethers
> Perfluorinated compounds
> Polycyclic aromatic hydrocarbons

pose a significant danger to fetuses during their development stages.

C) Vertically transmitted infections

These are infections caused by bacteria, viruses or parasites. They are passed from the mother to the child during the embryonic and fetal stages of pregnancy or during childbirth.

D) Malnutrition

This is a condition in which the body is deprived of specific nutrients. For example, a condition called *spina bifida* is caused by the lack of folic acid in the dietary habits of the mother during pregnancy.

E) Physical restraints

There is a condition called oligohydramnios. It describes the decrease of the volume of amniotic fluid which may be enough to significantly affect the morphogenesis of a fetus. This is an example of physical issues that may cause teratogenesis.

Exposure to these agents may explain why the disorder appears so early in childhood. Other causes examined pertain to environmental factors, but no theories are yet confirmed by research. On the contrary, some of them have been disproven and consequently dismissed.

The Mechanism

Asperger Syndrome, whatever the causes may be, seems to affect either the total or a major part of functional brain systems, instead of imposing a localized effect. Some researchers speculate that it may be necessary to separate the research for this specific disorder from the research conducted for the other disorders of the autistic spectrum, as they hypothesize that the mechanism is actually different here and it distinctively points to alterations in the brain development a short while after the embryo was conceived.

These alterations seem to be attributed to a migration of embryonic cells during the development of the fetus that is abnormal and affects the final structure of the brain and its connectivity. The theory supposes that there are high-level neural connections that are underperforming, which means that the synchronization between the functions, combined with the presence of excessive low-level processes, suffers greatly. This combination of factors is most likely the reason behind the delays in the cognitive functions and the loss of already attained skills.

The theory is supported by neuroanatomical studies, in association with the exposure to teratogens, which provide evidence that strongly support that the mechanism of alterations occurs in the development of the cerebellum right after the embryo's conception.

Other theories that have been developed and pertain to the mechanism behind Asperger's are the *weak central coherence theory*, which assumes that a limited ability to see the big picture is the cause behind the core disorder, and the *mirror neuron system theory,* which assumes that the alterations in the development stage interfere with the fundamental learning process of imitation and lead to the core feature of Asperger's, the impairment of social interaction.

Diagnosis

To find out if a child suffers from Asperger Syndrome, the standard criteria require the impairment of the social functions and interaction and the observance of stereotypic patterns of repetitive and restrictive behavior. This impairment should not extend to the language or other cognitive development. Furthermore, there has to be significant impairment in the everyday functioning of the child.

This usually happens between the ages of 4 and 11, and to make sure that the diagnosis is correct, the child should be assessed by a team of multidisciplinary observers that will render clinical judgment after the examination of three separate tests.

The examination should include:

➢ Evaluation of the neurological condition
➢ Evaluation of the genetics involved
➢ Cognitive tests

➢ Evaluation of the psychomotor functions
➢ Evaluation of the strengths and weakness in verbal and nonverbal communication
➢ Evaluation of the learning and knowledge acquisition style
➢ The ability for independent living

The relevant interviews include:

➢ The *Revised Autism Diagnostic Interview,* which is a semi-structured parent interview

➢ The *Autism Diagnostic Observation Schedule,* which is a conversation with the child and an interview based on play.

It is of utmost importance that the diagnosis occurs as early as possible and that there is no misdiagnosis involved. This latter case especially may cause additional problems, should medication be prescribed that will actually worsen the behavioral patterns.

Another reason for the earliest possible diagnosis is the fact that diagnosing adults is much more difficult. All the tests have been designed to address children and the symptoms exhibited change as the individual grows up. A very painstaking and time-consuming procedure would be required to diagnose an adult.

It would need to subject the person to a thorough clinical examination, and it would include a complete medical history as accumulated by the individual himself or herself. Additionally, interviews should be conducted with people who are familiar to and have detailed knowledge of the person's history and who can attest to behavioral patterns and changes.

Diagnosing Asperger's gets even more complicated in both children and adults as a differential diagnosis may be required which would consider a great number of affiliated disorders such as:

➢ Disorders of the schizophrenia spectrum
➢ O.C.D. (obsessive-compulsive disorder)
➢ Major depressive disorder
➢ Semantic pragmatic disorder
➢ Nonverbal learning disorder
➢ Tourette syndrome
➢ Stereotypic movement disorder
➢ Bipolar disorder
➢ Social and cognitive deficits that are produced by damage to the brain, including alcohol abuse

A major problem that has surfaced recently in reference to the diagnosis is that the cost involved and the difficulty of the screening process, along with the increasing popularity in using medication and the expansion of the benefits received, has produced an incentive to health providers to over-diagnose AS.

Screening

Before any child, adolescent or adult is put through the diagnosis process described above, they are put through a screening procedure which determines if any further testing is merited. This screening process begins with the parents.

They are typically able to identify even slight differences in the behavior of their child as early as the 30th month of age. It follows logically that they will require the opinion of a pediatrician or a general practitioner. They will determine, after a routine examination, if further investigation is needed. Should this be the case, a number of screening tools are available. These are:

➢ The Asperger Syndrome Diagnostic Scale (ASDS)

- The Childhood Autism Spectrum Test (CAST) (renamed from Childhood Asperger Syndrome Test)
- The Autism Spectrum Screening Questionnaire (ASSQ)
- The Krug Asperger's Disorder Index (KADI)
- The Gilliam Asperger's Disorder Scale (GADS)
- The Autism Spectrum Quotient (ASQ), which has different version for children, adolescents and adults

All of the above will indicate if there is an autism spectrum disorder but not which one. This is why the rest of the diagnostic process is necessary.

Prognosis

Twenty percent of people diagnosed with Asperger's in childhood may experience a lessening of the symptoms to the point that they no longer qualify as patients of the disorder when they reach adulthood. Another great percentage may experience a lessening of the symptoms, but will still be considered patients after the end of adolescence. In both cases, some social functions and communication skills may still be impaired.

There is no difference in the life expectancy of AS patients, but there is an increased chance that they will succumb to comorbid psychiatric conditions like depressive disorder and anxiety.

The most positive prognosis is that AS does not seem to affect the ability of some individuals to achieve, as amply displayed by the Nobel Prize awardee Vernon L. Smith.

The most critical aspect in the prognosis of Asperger Syndrome is the education of families and teachers. They can play the most significant role in helping their children (or students) and participate positively in the behavioral therapies. It is equally important that these people are able to cope with the situation, which may become extremely straining, especially the later the syndrome is diagnosed.

If the severity of the syndrome warrants such an action, it may be necessary to submit the children with AS to special educational facilities specially equipped and trained to handle their social and behavioral deficiencies.

Legal Implications

Another aspect to consider in Asperger's are the legal implications. Patients of the disorder may become subjects of exploitation by other individuals, or they may not be aware of the implications involved in their social actions. This is a concept that has caused much debate.

The aspies themselves (at least those with sufficient levels of cognitive abilities) do not consider Asperger's as a disorder but as a genetic difference, similar to homosexuality. If this notion prevails, then the aspies must be held responsible for all of their actions, regardless of their condition, in a court of law.

On the other hand, if the medical opinion prevails, aspies may stand to receive judgments of diminished capacity, when it comes to their actions, regardless of whether their condition allows them to have complete awareness of the consequences of what they have done.

In any case, Asperger Syndrome needs a lot more scientific studies and research that will provide a unified and definite answer as to the causes, the context and what must be done in order to satisfactorily remedy the situation. The aspies themselves may choose to reject this remedy if they are judged capable enough to decide for themselves, but the option must be available for those who choose not to suffer from society's misgivings, misconceptions and misunderstandings, or to be treated like curses or abominations.

Chapter 2: History

In the previous chapter, we discussed how Asperger Syndrome may not affect some of the abilities of certain individuals and their potential for great accomplishments. This is certainly the case with the Austrian pediatrician ***Hans Asperger***.

Hans Asperger was born on February 18, 1906, at Hausbrunn, which at the time belonged to the Austro-Hungarian Empire. He studied at the University of Vienna (where he also died on October 21, 1989, at the age of 74) and apart from his title as pediatrician, he was also a medical professor and a medical theorist.

According to some accounts of his personal history, he may have exhibited either some or all of the features of the syndrome during his childhood. These accounts tell of him being considered a lonely and remote child who had difficulty in finding friends. Asperger also had a great interest in the Austrian poet Franz Grillparzer. He was known to recite Grillperzer's poems to his classmates, even at times when they were quite uninterested in listening to them. In a Julius Caesar complex, Asperger would also refer to himself in the third person and frequently quoted himself repeatedly.

Asperger studied medicine under the teachings of Franz Hamburger and practiced his profession at the University Children's Hospital of Vienna. He spoke of Hamburger with great admiration and frequently mentioned that it was Hamburger who was responsible for his success as a pediatrician.

Asperger received his graduation discharge in 1931, became the director of the special education section of the same hospital in 1932, got married in 1935, and had five children.

These historical records indicate three very important things:

1) He did display some of the identifying symptoms of AS.
2) He had a normal and successful life which achieved greatness.
3) He would not have succeeded if it weren't for his teacher.

In 1944, as a pediatrician, he had four children under his supervision who displayed the social interaction difficulties and non-verbal communication impairments that became the cornerstone of the syndrome. At that time, he summed up his observations under what he called "*autistic psychopathy.*"

It was his important work that led to the name to the syndrome, even though it wasn't until fifty years later that the diagnosis began being standardized, and even though some of the processes differed significantly from his initial suggestions.

There was quite a lot of additional information pertaining to his work, but unfortunately, it was only published in the German language during wartime Germany. This made it difficult for Asperger to receive worldwide recognition. Furthermore, it's been said that he even went so far as to defend individuals suffering from autism against a country with a eugenics policy which would have demanded the extermination of such individuals.

Lorna Wing

In 1981, the English-speaking medical community was made aware of the Asperger Syndrome and its nuances through the publications of **Lorna Wing**. If there is anyone to thank for her work, which advanced the worldwide understanding of autism and developmental disorders that occur in childhood, it would be Wing.

Dr. Wing was a psychiatrist and a physician who studied Asperger's work and introduced the term *Asperger Syndrome* to the medical community. She was also involved in the founding of the English National Autistic Society. For her accomplishments she received the Order of the British Empire in 1994.

She was born Lorna Gladys Tolchard on October 7, 1928, at Gillingham Kent, UK, and she died at Kent at the age of 85 on Jun 6, 2014. She studied at the University College Hospital and, after her qualification as a psychiatrist, she was posted at Maudsley Hospital in London. She began her studies on childhood developmental disorders in 1959.

To document her research, Dr. Wing published a series of case studies in her 1981 introductory work *"Asperger Syndrome: a clinical account."* Provided below are details about some of the cases she studied. Knowing about these cases will help individuals understand what this syndrome is and how people that suffer from this syndrome react to things and live their lives.

Lorna Wing did a lot of research and studied a lot of individuals, so not all of them are addressed in this book. However, discussed below are three cases that seem different yet similar to each other.

Going through these, you will understand how the lives of individuals that suffer from AS are affected by people around them and, consequently, how they perceive other people and things. Additionally, these case studies note the opinions of other individuals, including the family of the sufferers, to help us understand how such individuals behave during childhood and how the people they are surrounded by are affected by this condition.

Case 1

This is a typical example of the syndrome. This example or case covers all the details about the individual from birth, through development and to finding the syndrome. This case should help readers to better understand this condition and be able to deal with people that suffer from this syndrome in a much more positive and helpful manner. Once you realize what aspies go through, you are in a better position to understand their pain.

At the age of 28, Mr. K.N. complained of shyness and nervousness. When he was a baby, he used to be happy and smiley and was rarely seen crying. His parents describe his early days as happy and sweet. He was a child who would calmly lie in his pram without crying and seem to be enjoying nature as it passed. Comparatively, his sister gave his mother more to worry about. While he was a silent toddler, his sister made all the noise in the house. He was different – he was always happy and actively avoided getting into fights and arguments with anyone, including other children who would take away his toys. He took a little longer than other kids to begin walking and was also a bit slow when it came to catching things, but this wasn't to a worrisome extent, according to his parents. To them, he seemed like any other kid, just a bit more restrained.

He started to talk when he was about one, which is the typical age when kids generally begin communicating. He would utter several broken words at this age, such as "mum" and "dad," etc.

(usual words for kids this age to say). However, an incident changed his habit. He stopped talking when he heard and saw a car crash, which left him devastated. He was silent for two long years and did not begin to speak again until he was three years of age. According to his parents, this was not something to worry about as they thought his understanding of speech patterns was similar to that of other children.

K. used to refer to himself in the third person until he reached the age of five, but he had a good understanding of grammar. Unlike most children his age, he would keep to himself and was not someone who would speak a lot. He wasn't very talkative and remained so even as he matured into an adult. He would only talk when he was spoken to and his answers were brief. He seemed to be disinterested in talking to people, and this was made more obvious from his monotonous voice and bored facial expressions. He just wasn't a social person.

As a child, he was close to his mother and did not have any friends outside of her because he was usually uncomfortable at school, getting bullied and teased. He was a shy individual who preferred to be alone and isolated. He, of course, had the desire to be social and make friends, but he did not succeed in doing so.

Growing up he was not good at games and had limited and ill-coordinated movements. He walked stiffly, without swinging his arm, and displayed signs of a good memory as he did well in subjects that required rote memorization. These subjects include the likes of Latin and history. He studied at a private school and was not good in doing creative tasks. He was a clumsy child and accordingly, the time he spent in the army was not enjoyable. He was there for a short period of time but did not take part in parades or marches, as he had poor coordination and could not do what was required of him. This is why he was quickly discharged.

K. was and is orderly in his regular routine and prefers to arrange his things himself. He is also not one to object to others or to changes that are imposed on him by others.

In his childhood, he was attracted by toy trains, cars and buses. He had a huge collection of such toys and was so much in love with them that he'd notice right away if any went missing. He preferred to play on his own and was rarely joined by others. He played with these toys until he was stopped from doing so. He'd indulge in self-play, using constructional kits for fun. This was his only "fun thing" as far as games are concerned, as he wasn't the kind of child who would go out and play with other kids. He was mostly home playing with his toys. His choice in toys displayed his interest in transport, which was something that stayed with him even into adulthood. He was immensely interested in vehicles and would often read books and novels related to cars and other forms of transportation. He was also a fan of watching shows related to cars. He would go on train trips with other enthusiasts just to experience the journey. His whole collection of books consisted of non-fiction that were related to cars, trains or other such vehicles. He had little to no interest in any other subject including stories and fantasy.

K. is now a clerk and has been employed for years, reportedly performing his services diligently. He says that he enjoys what he does. However, he says that he is well aware of his limits and would like to have friends and marry so that he could be happier and enjoy life to the fullest. He enjoys doing what he loves and also regularly writes columns for several magazines in order to help others who are dealing with similar problems. He was often called "shy," and many made him believe that this "shyness" was a problem that could be cured. These ideas were part of what motivated him to get in touch with a psychiatrist and hopefully find a solution to his problem.

He went to WAIS and was given an IQ test to judge his skills. The test included different types of sub-tests (non-verbal and verbal included) to judge his skills and rate him based on the results.

K. has been employed for many years in routine clerical work. He enjoys his job and his hobbies, but is very sad and anxious because he is aware of his own social ineptness. He writes many letters to advice columns in magazines, hoping for help with these problems. His concern over what he called his "shyness" finally made him ask for help from a psychiatrist. The test rated him "poor" particularly in the sub-test areas.

Case 2

This second case is similar to the first one, with major difference being that severe depression was also diagnosed during the early phases. The presence of depression makes this case unique and complex.

At the age of 24, Mr. L.P. was brought to a psychiatric hospital when he attempted to end his life. This suicide attempt, like other suicide attempts, was sad and had a long history behind it.

Mr. L.P. was a premature child (born about four weeks premature) and hence, had several issues at the beginning of his life, including feeding problems. However, this wasn't cause for any special concern as premature children usually have such problems and it is considered normal by many.

This example has several similarities with case no. 1 as here, too, the baby was placid, easy and quiet. He was rather unresponsive and would lie for hours without crying or making any sound.

He had a sister who made his parents realize that he was slower than other children of his age. He acquired self-care and motor skills, but a little later in development. However, this did not make his parents worried, even though his father did believe that something was wrong or missing in his son, but it was not deemed important enough for concern and hence, they did not seek any expert advice.

He started to speak at the age of three, which may be considered a little late but again, this did not worry his family much as he belonged to a bilingual family, and this attribute was considered the reason that he started to speak only later in life. Conversely, when he reached school-going age and was admitted to a school, he was able to create and speak long sentences to express himself and prove his points.

He had a habit of interpreting sentences in an odd manner and often spoke as if he were reading from a book. For example, if he heard a word like "independent," he assumed it meant that such a person was always in a pool's deep end. This habit of interpreting words incorrectly often caused him to fail to understand what was being explained to him. Apparently to compensate, he habitually asked questions again and again in order to make sense of what he was being told.

He did not take to jokes very lightly either and would often get offended as well. He'd rather stick to himself and not take part in conversations and when he did it would result in him asking questions repetitively as he usually failed to understand the conversations.

As a child, he was obedient and placid. He would generally sit idle and not do anything until he was instructed to or asked to join or take part in something. Unlike other children, he would just sit and rock rather than take part in imaginative play. Until he was fourteen, he had no friends and was rather lonely, even though he went to a normal school. In his early teenage years, he made two or three friends that were his companions for a while, but it wasn't long before he lost touch and was once again on his own. L. also does not have very fond memories of his school time, as he was usually bullied at school, and he considered himself rather unhappy during this period.

L. likes to take care of his possessions and keep them in a neat and proper manner. Also, he likes perfection as far as routine is concerned and will do things day in and day out in the same manner.

He has poor hand-eye coordination and hence, does not do well at games, especially games that require good motor skills. He is also seen with odd postures and expressions that look bewildered. Plus, he's in the habit of making gestures while speaking, but the gestures are considered inappropriate and jerky, especially when he is trying to express something. All of this, combined with his odd fashion sense, do not leave a very positive impact on people.

Shortcomings aside, he has an excellent memory which allows him to score well on exams, especially in subjects that required rote memorization. His hobby is playing chess, and he is very good at it. He can play for hours and usually win matches. His other hobbies include reading books related to chemistry and physics. He has also memorized a great number of scientific facts. He has a detailed interest in time and can be seen wearing a number of watches (usually two). These watches generally show different times (local and GMT).

As evident in such cases, his biggest problem is his social ineptitude. His audience generally gets bored of him rather quickly. He is also uncomfortable when he is surrounded by people and ends up acting childish and making remarks he shouldn't make. Like mentioned in case 1, he is well aware of his shortcomings but hasn't been able to do much about it. He is trying to acquire skills to overcome his deficiency but nothing has helped yet. However, he is a good human being, is very kind to others, and does his best to help people. If he finds out someone is ill or in trouble, he makes it a point to show concern and help the individual if he can.

He lives in a hotel and works as a clerk. His parents refrained from seeking psychiatric help for him as a child, but he hired the services of several psychiatrists once he reached adolescence as he was quite aware of his inabilities and wanted to overcome them.

He reports getting worried when thinking about sex and other intimate, interpersonal aspects of life. He also reported having lost sleep due to changes in his work routine, and all this prodded him to seek psychiatric help. The third time he sought psychiatric help was after a suicide attempt, which was again apparently due to changes at work that affected him to such a degree that he decided to end his life.

He is a good swimmer, and this maybe the reason why he is still alive, as he once attempted to kill himself by drowning but stayed afloat due to his ability to swim. Other suicide attempts include trying to strangle himself, but again without success. In his own words, he says that this is due to the fact that he is not a very practical person.

At admission (after the suicide attempt), he looked disheartened and shattered and spoke with broken speech. He did give replies that were true and relevant to the context, though not always related to the question that was asked. There were also long gaps between his words. For example, when he was questioned about what kind of a relationship he shares with his dad, L. replied "My father and I get on well. He is a man who likes gardening."

L. believes that all of the blame for his failures falls on himself. He thinks of himself as a person who is unpleasant and not liked by anyone. He also thinks he lacks the ability to manage his own life.

He says that whatever people think of him may be right. He has heard people call him stupid and a "chemistry fanatic." However, some questioning and observation showed that these claims were nothing more than misinterpretations of some conversations he had overheard.

These multiple suicide attempts have been attributed to anxiety (in the case of the first two), schizophrenia (the third time), and finally Asperger syndrome that was further complicated due to the prevalence of depression and anxiety.

L. has a large vocabulary that helped him score an average range on the WAIS.

Case 3

This third case study is different from the two mentioned earlier, as in this case the abnormality was recognized in infancy. This case of B.H. is of value due to this reason.

B.H. is about 10 years of age and, as a newborn, was delivered by forceps. He is said to have difficulty with breathing and was in the special care unit for two weeks after his birth. B.H. was a large and placid baby, who like the other two cases mentioned earlier, would silently lie for hours without crying or making any other noise. He was also a very still baby who'd rarely use hand movements or make gestures. Unlike the other two cases, his mother was concerned for him, mainly due to the birth complications and behavior issues that he had.

He started to utter words when he was about 11 months old and would speak fluently when he was about fourteen months old. His language was broken, but he could speak the way a fourteen-month-old child is expected to. He did not make any effort to crawl, however, but suddenly started walking when he was a year and a half old, and only started to crawl after this.

The language he spoke was, to an extent, the "baby language" that stayed with him until he was three years of age and this is when he started to speak clearly and to gain an understanding of speech and words. His expressions showed that he had difficulty in comprehending sentences. Conversing is something his parents believe he learnt from television as it wasn't taught to him by them. His comprehension stayed poor even when he was five years old; at around this time he could read really well (better than most children of his age), but he had issues comprehending things.

He was a gentle child who did not give any trouble to his parents and was rarely demanding. He would usually stay quiet and did not show much emotion regarding any changes around him, even when they were forced on him by others.

Like the above two cases, B.H. didn't develop any imaginative pretend play either. When he reached the age of six, he started to take interest in different types of vehicles, including cars and airplanes. He would watch cars and planes and was keen to know more about them. He also used to play with such toys, but these activities never involved other children and he preferred to keep to himself.

He has a phobia (climbing) and some coordination issues that cause him trouble with laces and buttons. Like other individuals suffering from this syndrome, he appears fairly clumsy.

B.H. goes to a special school where he had issues settling in at the beginning. He did not initially mingle with his peers and would remain by himself. He also had issues when he was told he'd have to obey the teacher and do as he was instructed. However, gradually he started to fit in, and he also began to interact with others, but in a rather naïve fashion. In addition, he is also said to have issues in following the rules when he's playing any sort of game.

B.H. speaks with an accent that is different from locals. He is also imaginative when it comes to making sentences. For example, he'd say, "I have a temporary loss of knitting" when he had a hole in his sock. This is thought to be the impact of learning through television, as a number of his phrases are odd and adopted.

B.H. has tried to socialize with others but has not been able to learn the art. He is well aware of others' criticisms though. He was tested when he was seven years of age and did well on some tests, including word recognition, but was ranked poorly on comprehension.

Modifications of Asperger's account

The author has mentioned quite a few additional points in the history of this syndrome that were not originally recorded by Asperger. These points can be elicited from suitable questioning of the individuals living around the sufferers, such as parents and siblings.

The signs include:

➢ During the first few years, there may be a lack of the regular interest and enjoyment in human interaction.

➢ During the first few years, babbling may be limited in quality and quantity.

➢ During the first few years, the individual may not pay much attention to surroundings or things that are happening around him or her.

➢ During the first few years, the child may not bring his or her toys to visitors or parents.

In general, these signs basically mean that the child in early years shows little to no interest in interacting with others. This may be realized by noticing that the child does not speak to anyone using either words or gestures. The child is also generally less reactive and is rarely seen reacting to jokes or comments (laughing, smiling, etc.) in comparison to normal children of this age.

Another very important factor is imaginative play, which is common among children, but individuals or children suffering from AS do not usually take part in pretend play. Conversely, those that do take part in such play usually have the "play" confined to only a few themes with little or no variation.

In addition, this play usually does not involve other children unless the partner is willing to play "by the rules," or to follow the pattern set by the individual in question. In some cases, this "pretend play" continues in adult life as well and takes the individual to a world that is nonexistent. This is discussed further in the case history of "Richard L." (*Bosch, 1962*).

The author also disagrees with quite a few claims and findings made by Asperger. Basically, there are two points that are of importance here. These are:

➢ Asperger states that such individuals are able to speak before they are able to walk. In his words, they have "an especially intimate relationship with language" and "highly sophisticated linguistic skills." However, new reports suggest that a great number of people that suffer from this syndrome begin to walk at the normal age but started to speak a little later. This point was heavily emphasized by Van Krevelen (1971)

➢ The second point of differentiation is in the fact that Asperger believed individuals that suffered from this condition were creative with a lot of original ideas. However, as evident from the case studies above, such individuals are believed to have a good memory, but their creativity is very limited and narrowed to a single point of interest. This clarification has also been verified now with the help of several tests that highlight a lack of creativity and originality in such individuals. Additionally, Asperger was of the idea that individuals suffering with his syndrome were of very high intelligence. However, he refrained from quoting results of any tests to support his claim. Though the studies and test results have proven that these individuals have good memory, they cannot be called "intelligent," as they are usually only able to score well in tests or subjects that require rote memorization and they lack the ability to do well in subjects that require dynamic intelligence or comprehension skills.

Another very important point that must be highlighted here is that the individuals Asperger studied are today described by experts of being in need of psychiatric help. A total of nine students were school dropouts and did not pursue any further education. Out of these nine, only three were able to get and retain their jobs, another three lost their jobs, while the remaining three were not able to acquire any jobs.

Differential Diagnosis

Like any other disease, the diagnosis of Asperger's Syndrome can be difficult at times, especially in people that show signs of abnormal or different behavior but do not necessarily suffer from this condition.

Those with years of experience in the field can usually easily recognize cases with the use of their experience and other tools used to diagnose this syndrome.

The latest research shows that the syndrome mixes into different clinical pictures like eccentric normality. This is the reason why no clear cut-off points have been identified yet and will not be established until and unless we are able to know more about the underlying pathology. In order to have a correct diagnosis and to be able to reach a solid point, one needs every detail, including birth complications (if any), developmental history, behavioral reports from childhood and through development, and a present clinical picture. If any of these items are missing, it may be difficult to diagnose this disease properly.

Normal Variant of Personality

Believe it or not, one of the main issues with the diagnosis of this disease is that a great number of features that characterize Asperger syndrome are found in the normal population as well. Though these signs are present, however, the degrees to which they exist differ, and this is the main aspect that is used to diagnose this syndrome.

All people are different, and some are even antisocial. As evident from the studies and cases mentioned above, one of the main signs of an individual suffering from this disease is the fact that he or she shies away from social interaction, as he or she may not comfortable or not know how to behave in public. Conversely, we have to understand that there are individuals who are antisocial, but this does not mean that they are suffering from Asperger's Syndrome.

The skills possessed by individuals also differ. Likewise, there's a broad distribution of general motor skills. Many individuals have some unique and weird hobbies that they wish to pursue with enthusiasm. These include collecting objects like soaps, stamps, glass bottles, or/and railway engine numbers. These people are normal individuals and their hobbies are also socially accepted.

Asperger, too, in 1979, mentioned that, "the capacity to withdraw into an inner world of one's own special interests is available in a greater or lesser measure to all human beings." He emphasized that the presence of this ability maybe a sign of intelligence and is usually seen in the scientists and artists who are creative.

There are many people who may show symptoms common among the individuals suffering from Asperger's Syndrome, but they are not necessarily suffering from this condition. It is very important to be able to differentiate between an individual with this condition and an individual who merely has such quirks and is living a complex life, albeit away from society. The main difference is that with a normal individual, these decisions to be unsocial or have complex and unique hobbies are most likely due to past social experiences. However, someone suffering from AS does not make the decision to behave in such a way, nor does he have past social experiences to blame.

Other issues or characteristics that are found in normal individuals include:

➢ Excellent rote memory

➢ Eidetic imagery

➢ Pedantic speech

However, just the presence of the above mentioned qualities is enough to diagnose a person as an Asperger's patient. Having a good rote memory is a sign of Asperger's syndrome, but it does not mean that only those suffering from this syndrome are skilled in this department. In the same way, artists often have eidetic memory which they use to their advantages. Lastly, pedantic speech maybe caused by several issues. All these points are just signs and symptoms of the Asperger's Syndrome, and their mere presence doesn't mean one has AS; these symptoms are not exclusive to aspies. It is important not to consider someone a patient just because these traits are seen in the individual. This is when the diagnosis phase, a very complex phase, comes into play. Calling someone a patient without being sure may have a very negative impact on that individual and may negatively impact his or her life.

Schizoid Personality

The lack of single-mindedness, empathy, odd communication, over-sensitivity, and social isolation are signs that are related to the Asperger's syndrome. However, these features are also a part of the definition of schizoid personality (Wolff & Chick, 1980).

Experts believe that there is a strong connection between AS and schizoid personality. However, the main question here is if this grouping can add something to our understanding and is it of any worth. This question and classification are discussed below in detail.

Schizophrenia

One of the biggest issues in the diagnosis of Asperger Syndrome is that it is often misdiagnosed, as its symptoms are quite similar to that of schizophrenia. Due to this fact, AS adults are quite often misdiagnosed as schizophrenic. The differential diagnosis of this disease is discussed in detail (J.K. Wing, 1978), but the main issue that arises in the diagnostics is the fact that schizophrenia is not thoroughly defined. Schizophrenia has several loose definitions, and due to this ambiguity, parallels are sometimes drawn with Asperger's syndrome.

If one accepts a loose definition of the disease that only highlights characteristics like speech disorders and social withdrawal, then one may include Asperger's syndrome in the same group of disorders as schizophrenia.

But again, the question is if there are any advantages of doing so. A lack of social interaction and poor speech may have varied causes, thus, the diagnosis of schizophrenia covers a number of situations which seem to have very little in common.

Careful scrutiny of speech in Asperger's syndrome shows dissimilarity from thought blocking described in 1922 by Bleuler. In cases of Asperger's syndrome, speech maybe broken or slow with tangential or irrelevant replies to what is asked, but these issues may be due to a propensity to get stuck in conversational grooves.

Utterances are, however, always logical, even in cases where they're not related to what's asked. A good example is of a man, when asked a question about organized charities replied, "They do things for unfortunate people. They provide wheelchairs, stilts and round shoes for people with no feet." There is an obvious contrast between the pedantic methodology found in the syndrome and the vagueness of schizophrenia.

The schizophrenia diagnosis can and should be used strictly. It needs to be confined to individuals that have, sometime in their life, shown the symptoms explained by Schneider in 1971.

The main differentiation between AS and schizophrenia lies on the precise definition of the phenomena. Unless sufferers have superimposed schizophrenia, those with Asperger's syndrome do not usually experience thought insertion or substitution, thought echo, voices in the head, and/or thought broadcast. Unlike those with schizophrenia, aspies also don't report feeling that any external force is trying to exert control over their emotions, behavior or will. This forced aspect is, instead, one of the major signs of schizophrenia.

In the case of L.P. discussed above, when questioned if he had any such experiences, he said, "I believe such things to be impossible."

During examination, it is essential to know that the ability to comprehend abstract concepts is weakened in people with Asperger's syndrome. Some individuals are in the habit of saying "yes" to whatever they're asked, as this is their way to cope and stop conversations, making the truth difficult to find and diagnose. This is why case history is important. Also, some patients have been found to borrow replies from other patients and use them when they're asked a question.

Other Psychotic Syndromes

Individuals suffering from Asperger's syndrome often have the propensity to over-generalize things as they are extra sensitive. They may also react to being made fun of, or if they feel that they're being made fun of, and thus their condition maybe incorrectly diagnosed as paranoid psychosis.

Several individuals tend to hallucinate and live in their own imaginary world. People with AS are often believed to be delusional by others. A very famous case is of a boy who had the notion that Batman was actually real and would one day arrive to take him on one of his crime fighting ventures. This, of course, made no logical sense, but no explanation could convince the boy that

Batman was not real nor was he ever going to appear. This is an example of a person being delusional or hallucinating, but a better term for it is having an "over-valued idea." However, this is not something that one can use in the diagnosis of AS or any other condition because such ideas are found in dozens of psychiatric conditions.

In addition to the above mentioned points, a number of other issues may be present, such as social withdrawal, odd postures and echopraxia. These conditions, like the above mentioned "over-valued ideas," though a sign of Aspergers's syndrome, cannot be definitive in helping the diagnosis as they're present in several other mental conditions (like encephalitis).

Obsessional Neurosis

One of the main signs of Asperger's syndrome is that the patient takes part in one repetitive task. However, the awareness of this illogicality, a characteristic of obsessional neurosis, isn't found in individuals with Apserger's syndrome. In order to diagnose the syndrome properly, it would be wise to examine the relationship of Asperger syndrome to obsessional personality, post-encephalitic obsessional conditions, and obsessional illness.

Affective Conditions

The lack of expressions, quietness, and social withdrawal in Asperger's syndrome may lead to one interpreting it as a depressive illness, and hence leading to a misdiagnosis. Distress and/or shyness in conditions when one is away from recognizable surroundings could lead to a person being anxious and help with the diagnosis. Also, when talking about an exciting, imaginary location, the condition of hypomania may see more relevant. Yet, background details and clinical pictures should help in the correct diagnosis.

Major difficulties arise when these illnesses are imposed on Asperger's syndrome. In such a situation, more time and data is required because doctors have to do a double diagnosis, both on the patient's present state and the past state in the light of all the available facts.

Early Childhood Autism

Asperger in his studies found a number of similarities between Asperger's syndrome and early childhood autism. Nonetheless, according to his conclusion the two were very different as he considered autism to be a psychotic process, while in his opinion, his syndrome was a personality trait that was stable. However, since not much is discussed about the two, there is a need to study them further to be able to reach such conclusions.

Experts like Wolff & Barlow (1979) and Van Krevelen (1971) agree with Asperger and accept that Asperger's syndrome is different from early childhood autism. However, the latest research shows that the two have more in common than initially believed.

Some important points are:

> A child suffering from autism is indifferent and aloof to the world, at least when he is young. However, comparatively, the child with Asperger's syndrome is seen making passive, one-sided approaches which may also be inappropriate.

> A child suffering from autism has abnormal or delayed speech, and may even be mute. Comparatively, a child that has Asperger's syndrome can learn to

speak with proper grammar and vocabulary. Conversely, it should be mentioned that a child with AS may have a proper vocabulary, but he or she may not be able to speak socially and could end up uttering words that are inappropriate or irrelevant, as such children have issues comprehending sentences.

➢ An autistic child may not use gestures to emphasize a message. However, in case of Asperger's syndrome, individuals do use gestures (though mostly inappropriate) to accompany words. In both these situations, monotonous vocal intonation is a leading characteristic.

➢ A child with autism develops repetitive and stereotyped routines involving people or objects. They may, for example, always set toys or other things in the same arbitrary order or insist that everyone in a room sits in a specific manner, no matter where or with whom. Conversely, in case of Asperger's syndrome, individuals usually become immersed in or obsessed with learning more about facts that they already find interesting (science, etc.).

> Irregular answers to sensory input – like indifference, fascination and distress – are some of the main characteristics of childhood autism. These are linked with a lower mental age. These signs are not common in older autistic people and are not described as typical of Asperger's syndrome either.

> This comparison does not lie in case of coordination and motor balancing skills. Generally, children that are autistic have no difficulty in balancing and climbing. However, in comparison, those with Asperger's syndrome suffer from hand-eye coordination issues and have poor motor skills.

In 1962, Bosch reached the conclusion that both these instances are variants of one condition. Unlike Van Krevelen and Asperger, most believe that in practice these two conditions do not differentiate into two different groups. However, both of these conditions must be studied further before scientists reach a conclusion regarding their categorization.

Aetiology and Pathology

In 1944, Asperger stated that his syndrome could be genetically transmitted. He believed this to be true because he noticed that the characteristics occurred more commonly in families, especially those families in which the fathers had this syndrome.

However, research about this aspect is ongoing, and it is too early to reach a conclusion, though there are signs that hint towards Asperger being right in his claim.

The syndrome is usually found in individuals with a history of post-, pre-, or peri-natal conditions, like anoxia at birth. These conditions are thought to damage the cerebral lobe in the brain and may give rise to Asperger's syndrome. It has also been proven that this syndrome may be due to an organic deficiency in brain functions.

Other factors include child-rearing methods that diverge from the norm. Additionally, emotional reasons are thought to play a part in the presence of this syndrome, especially in cases where someone in the family, particularly the father, mother and/or brothers and sisters show similar peculiarities to that of the patient. However, this theory is nothing more than a claim right now, and there is little to no evidence to prove this claim correct. One would need very thorough epidemiological studies to be able to reach a definite conclusion regarding this theory.

The findings of Dr. Wing compelled *Uta Frith* to translate all of Hans Asperger's work from German to English in 1991. *Gillberg and Gillberg* and *Szatmari et al.* in 1989 outlined a set of diagnostic criteria, and Asperger Syndrome became a standard diagnosis in 1992.

However, this was reversed in the latest edition of the Diagnostic and Statistical Manual of Mental Disorders in 2013, and the diagnosis of Asperger Syndrome is no longer differentiated. Instead, it's included under the general diagnosis of autism spectrum disorder, though on a different scale of severity from other autism conditions.

Chapter 3: Effects of the Syndrome on Social Interaction

We have repeatedly mentioned in the previous chapters the problems, inadequacies and difficulties exhibited by the patients with Asperger Syndrome in reference to their social functions, skills and interactions. It's now time to take a closer look at them.

One thing to always keep in mind is that the social interaction problems pertain to the views of the people around the patients and not to the patients themselves. Just as some people feel quite comfortable being around other people, aspies feel comfortable being left alone and at liberty to carry on with their daily routines and interests without outside interference.

One of the main arguments used by the supporters of the notion that those who exhibit the symptoms of the syndrome and present no danger to themselves or others should be considered as merely "different" and not as patients is that the obsession to force aspies into acquiring these social interaction skills is an invasion of privacy. This policy aims not to benefit the aspies but the rest of the social network.

The latest studies on the subject found that both views are actually incorrect. People with AS **want** to interact socially like anyone else. They **want** to acquire friendships as much as anyone else. So it is wrong to assume that they want to be left alone, but it is also wrong to say that teaching them what they need to know about social interaction is an invasion of privacy.

If someone wants to interact socially and have friends, there are some rules and protocols involved that must be respected. When this someone has no knowledge or perception of these rules and protocols, he or she may feel and act out of context. Thus, they need to be shown these rules and protocols.

The first issue that seriously impacts people with AS, not so much for them as for the people of their immediate environment, is the apparent lack of empathy. People who do not know that this person on the other side of the social circumstance suffers from Asperger's get incensed when it comes to the lack of attention they are receiving. Quite commonly, aspies show almost no signs of empathy either towards or against the speaker's side of the story.

When people talk to someone about their problems, their dreams, and their opinions, they expect a response from those to whom they talk. When they do not receive an appropriate response, they lash out against the person on the other side of the conversation, without considering that they may be facing a person who is suffering from a disorder. As a result of this disorder, the person may have no interest in listening to anyone's problems, dreams or opinions. They also do not know how to respond to what the other person is saying to them.

This dilemma leads to difficulty in acquiring friendships, failure to enjoy shared activities in which others participate, and failure to celebrate achievements of other people. This deficiency brings forth one of the main issues of social interaction, which is the "give-and-take" mechanic, or, more scientifically, the ability to demonstrate emotional reciprocity.

The rest of the characteristics, like impaired nonverbal communication skills, clumsy or non-existent body posture or gesturing, and a lack of facial expression, are all results of these two basic concepts – empathy and emotional reciprocity.

A crucial distinction must be made at this point. ***Nonverbal communication is not the same as body language.*** Nonverbal communication is a concept that supersedes and encompasses body language. The definition of nonverbal communication is the process of communication that uses wordless signals.

This includes kinesics (the body language), paralanguage (vocal expressions and qualities), haptics (touch), proxemics (concepts of space and distance), and aspects of the physical environment and appearance. It also includes chronemics, the concepts behind the use of time within a communication, which is usually overlooked by doctors and researchers alike.

For a trained eye, a lot more can be said through nonverbal communication than with a verbal one. There is an entire science called *the study of micro-expressions*. The professionals of this discipline study the facial expressions in split second intervals to determine characteristics or emotions that are not present in speech. This science is used extensively in politics to determine if a politician is lying or has something to hide.

While not everyone has studied and immersed themselves in the study of micro-expressions, some aspects are instinctively observed, as they warn others about the negative feelings of the person displaying them. It is well-known throughout the world that avoiding eye-contact means a person is telling a lie or has something to hide.

The lack of facial expressions and displays of emotions is not so much a problem of showing emotions as it as a problem of not being able to understand how others feel. It is a natural tendency of the human being to trust feelings more than words. When not perceiving or receiving these expressions of feelings, people are less likely to trust the speaker. Consequently, we tend not to like the person who shows no feelings.

But these are not the only problems that pertain to impaired social interactions. Another basic impairment is the frequent urge of an aspie to engage in a monologue. In this monologue he or she talks constantly about a certain topic in a long-winded speech. During the process, he or she does not interpret or understand that the listener(s) may wish to end the conversation or change the topic. They also fail to recognize and often misinterpret the reactions and feelings of the listener to said monologue. This has also been incorrectly interpreted as insensitiveness or as a disregard of the other people's feelings.

Since the syndrome falls under the general category of mental disorders, in the beginning there were some hypotheses stating that aspies were prone to violent behavior and criminal acts. All the relevant studies dismissed these hypotheses as the findings showed that they are more often the victims rather than the victimizers. All of the cases which included aspies in violent and criminal activities occurred by perpetrators who were suffering from a co-existing disorder in the psychiatric range, like the schizoaffective one.

Further studies and research on the effects of AS on the social interaction sphere, showed that in many cases, children and adolescents suffering from this syndrome can behave normally and exhibit regular social interactions and functionality in a closed environment with controlled conditions. The same aspies, when they were taken out into the real world, where the circumstances are not controlled and are more fluid, reverted to their original behaviors and difficulties.

When this happened, the subjects' analysis and observations led them to adopt a rigid behavioral guideline and to apply what they had learned in awkward ways. This further augmented the problem as the more failed social encounters they had, the more their behavior became rigid and unchangeable.

A side effect of these social encounters may result in an aspie developing a condition called *selective mutism*. This happens when, within a social environment, they do not talk at all to most of the people present but focus and talk excessively and exclusively to people that they think they can trust or that they like.

This makes them vulnerable to manipulation and should such trust be abused, then they stop addressing other people altogether. They will speak only when they are addressed directly and only about topics in which they are interested. It would not be surprising then, if, in a social environment, they withdrew to a location where they thought that no one would notice and occupied themselves with a hobby or an interest.

Because of their idiosyncratic behavior and the failure of other people to understand their situation, aspies may not respond well to notions such as sarcasm, banter or metaphors. Even jokes are sometimes taken seriously and they may feel insulted without understanding the reason behind the insult.

It is unknown at this time why aspies tend to be especially gifted in mathematics and spatial skills. (Some researchers attribute this peculiarity to nature's tendency to achieve "balance" in every situation.) This actually results in more problems, as these children may consider what they are taught in school as ordinary and mundane, while they themselves have progressed far beyond. Inevitably, this results in problems with the teachers and, later on, with figures of authority.

The last issue to consider in reference to the effects of the syndrome on social skills is that concerning marriage and intimate relationships. In these instances, steps must be taken to remedy the situation for the benefit of the aspie. A lack of empathy and emotional reciprocity is, by default, the opposite of the feelings required for such relationships.

How can someone who doesn't even understand what love is, fall in love with someone else? And how can any "someone else" accept the fact that their partner may show no interest, no love, no empathy and no emotions in return?

Such issues are the basis and the focus of the behavioral therapies that are applied to aspies in an attempt to improvement of their social skills. They *can* live a normal life, but they have to learn how.

Chapter 4: Effects of the Syndrome on Behavior and Interests

One of the most important indications that someone is suffering from Asperger Syndrome is their behavior. This is the one symptom that is always present in all cases, and it has to do with the activities and interests which are pursued with abnormal focus and intensity. Aspies devise a daily routine and then stick to it invariably, and they tend to occupy themselves with a specific topic, a specific issue or a specific object.

At this point, it should be stated that aspies can go through their routines and their interests without necessarily understanding why they do it, or even what it is they are doing. They can collect images of stars, for example, without knowing any additional information about the subject. They do it just because they like the pictures. They can even memorize numbers without even the most basic of understanding of mathematics.

This process usually begins around the age of six. In the beginning, they may be involved in a broader spectrum of interests, but as time passes by, and even though these interests may change, the focus becomes narrower and the interests become more unusual. Sometimes this display overwhelms the aspie's family to the point that they become completely immersed.

A problem in this case is that it's normal, to some extent, for a child to become focused on a specific topic from time to time, and this obsession may pass undetected for some time. This is why it is most imperative to pay attention to body language.

The successful diagnosis of AS includes the behavioral and interest patterns as its core part. This part includes the observation of flapping and twisting, other movements of the hands, and complex movements of the entire body. When these movements are repeated in a fashion which seem more prolonged, natural and symmetrical than the simple nervous tic would, it is often an indication of the presence of Asperger's.

To better understand what the observation should be looking for, nervous tics are much faster, involuntary, and without rhythm or symmetry. The movements of the hands and the body of a child suffering from AS are longer, they seem voluntary and ritualistic, and they have rhythm and symmetrical patterns.

Another integral part of the diagnosis of AS is the lack of imagination. A child is normal when he or she plays "as if." Scientifically, this is called imaginative play: a boy pretends that the car he is playing with is the famous Batmobile, or a girl pretends that her doll is a princess.

Children that suffer from the syndrome prefer non fictitious activities and interests, and they have no wish to watch or listen to fairy tales. If a boy plays with a car, that's what he plays with, a car. Not a Batmobile or a Formula 1. If this kind of behavior is noticed, it is a most definite indication of Asperger's.

Stereotypy is defined as a repetitive motion, stance or sound. It can be displayed as simple motions, like body rocking, or through more complex ones, like self-caressing or marching in place. It is considered a standard issue in people suffering from intellectual disabilities such as Asperger's.

Stereotyped behavior does not necessarily mean that the child suffers from Asperger's. It is a clear indication only. It must be verified by the appropriate doctors, as it has been linked with other medical conditions like tardive dyskinesia, stereotypic movement disorder and some types of schizophrenia.

Stereotypy is also associated with frontotemporal lobar degeneration, which is pathological and not psychological or mental and which occurs in people suffering from frontotemporal dementia. An appropriate examination should uncover an atrophy in the frontal and temporal lobes of the brain while the parietal and occipital ones are left intact. Asperger's is suspected when these issues are **not** shown in the tests.

In all four types of autism, stereotypy is called stimming, as it is hypothesized that it is performed as a self-stimulus of the senses, rather than as a method of expression or counterbalance, as it is in other conditions. This is another one of the reasons that the diagnosis must be correct.

If an aspie is given medication that is recommended for schizophrenics, for example, then his or her behavior will get worse. He or she will also have to undergo a different set of cognitive therapies which will actually do very little to improve the condition.

At this time, we need to address another side of stereotypy. The term also means assigning traits to a class of people and assuming that these traits are always there. Let's discuss what the typical stereotypes about people with Asperger Syndrome are.

➢ They are supposedly unable to do things that require social interaction.
➢ They dislike eye contact.
➢ They dislike using the telephone and prefer indirect or person-to-person means of communication.
➢ They get disoriented and have trouble hearing in social situations where there is a lot of people and noise.
➢ They are easily depressed.
➢ Small talk and intimate banter is out of their league.
➢ They assume that all comments or remarks must be responded to.
➢ Most of the time, they do not care what other people think.

> Most of the time, they cannot read the body language of other people.

> They may feel rejected and regard themselves as failures if a project or an idea they consider as important receives a mixed or lukewarm response.

> Their method of interaction makes others angry.

> Facing a frustrating situation, they often respond angrily.

> In conversation, they are sometimes tactless or divergent and their language is inappropriate.

> When they talk about a topic, they talk forever without pause.

> If they are asked a question that is difficult to answer, they remain silent.

This is how the rest of the world has **stereotyped** people with AS. Half of the above are myths, some more are greatly exaggerated and only a few are actually true, falling within the symptoms that have already been described.

This is a clear and indisputable indication that while the general population may have knowledge of the term "Asperger Syndrome," they have insufficient knowledge of the symptoms and how people with AS actually behave. This means that there has to be a campaign of information and education on the subject.

Another aspect of the stereotyping of the aspies as a category of people, is that all the above are **negative**. If the general population wants to attribute stereotyped traits to aspies, why not attribute the following:

- ➢ Their auditory perception may make them the best sound engineers and quite eligible to work in a recording studio.
- ➢ Their sensitivity to taste and texture may make them exceptional gastronomes and food critics.
- ➢ Their eye for detail may be quite beneficial to photography, drawing and assisting architects and artists.
- ➢ They have no sexism or racism issues.
- ➢ They are very sensitive to disadvantaged people like themselves and could contribute as mediators or arbiters in disputes.
- ➢ There is extensive documentation of great innovation and invention from people with AS, not only in tangible subjects, but also in ideas and story-telling.

- They are relatively incapable of dishonesty, of lying and of many other negative traits of mankind.
- Their memory retention may actually be quite exceptional, especially with numbers, historical facts and past situations.
- They may have great powers of deduction which make them ideal for crime investigators.
- They may have difficulties in acquiring friendships, but they are very loyal friends themselves.

The problem of societal acceptance of the aspies will be further discussed in the following chapters. As a prelude to that discussion, it is worth mentioning that if one was to distance oneself and conduct a study as an outside observer, he would notice that if a balance was used to weigh the positives and the negatives of people with AS, the scale would tilt in favor of the positives.

Chapter 5: Effects of the Syndrome on Speech and Language

In some cultures, to indicate that something is extremely obvious, they use the following joke:

"What meows on the roof and is not a dog that also learns foreign languages?"

It is obvious that the answer to this question is "a cat." In the case of Asperger's, unfortunately, the aspie may be the dog that tries to learn foreign languages. As stated in relevant studies, in many cases linguistic communication for people with AS is an attempt at mimicry without any understanding of the underlying nuances.

The concept of language is the vocal expression of meanings and feelings. The correct use of language means that the person who is speaking interprets the meanings and feelings of his own brain and matches them to the appropriate words in an orderly fashion.

Aspies usually do not experience delays in the acquisition of language skills, and their speech patterns are quite normal. But they may *seem* to be atypical, in that they incorporate any or all of the following in their use of language:

- ➢ Verbosity
- ➢ Pedantism
- ➢ Literal interpretation
- ➢ Lack of nuance comprehension
- ➢ Abrupt transitions
- ➢ Use of metaphors that make sense only to the speaker
- ➢ Formal or idiosyncratic speech

This atypical use of language most often results from problems in the auditory perception of the aspie. While the sounds will reach the brain, due to the abnormalities of the brain functions, the individual will have difficulty in correctly interpreting and understanding the sounds he or she hears, especially those that pertain to speech. These auditory perception deficits may also result in peculiar uses of loudness, pitch, prosody, intonation and rhythms of speech patterns.

For an accurate diagnosis of the syndrome, three aspects are needed: prosody that is poor, circumstantial and tangential speech, and marked verbosity. These are indicated by the following factors:

➤ Limited range of intonation
➤ Unusually fast, jerky and loud speech
➤ Speech that may sound incoherent
➤ Monologues on topics that result in the boredom of the listener
➤ Speech that fails to provide context for comments
➤ Speech that fails to suppress internal thoughts
➤ Failure to understand if the listener is interested in the topic or not
➤ Failure to understand if the listener is engaged in the conversation
➤ Failure to conclude or make a point
➤ Disregard of the listener's attempts to elaborate on the topic
➤ Disregard of the listener's attempts to change the topic

Hans Asperger called the children under his care "little professors." This was due to their literal usage of language. Aspies seem to have difficulty in understanding and using *figurative speech*. Consequently, expressions of humor, irony, sarcasm and teasing seem not only to escape them completely, but also to insult them.

Especially in the case of humor, aspies may understand the cognitive basis but cannot understand the concept of humor being used as a means to share enjoyment with other people. Strangely, while the evidence for the lack of humor appreciation is strong, there have been reports of humor in aspies that challenge some of the theories about the psychological status of the people that exhibit the symptoms of AS.

Sometimes aspies will display **echolalia**. The term is the same as **echologia** or **echophrasia**. This is the automatic or delayed repetition of speech that the aspie hears from another person. The relevant studies conducted in the 1980s, theorized that they do this in an attempt to communicate through imitative behavior.

The practice can be considered an attempt at the superficial processing of linguistic skills or at the deeper level processing of contextual information. It may also be an attempt to learn.

When an aspie repeats a phrase he or she has heard on the TV or radio, a favorite script or a parental instruction, he or she may be attempting to process this information for the purpose of understanding the meanings and thus becoming able to use them later on in discussions.

While this intention may work and the aspie may memorize the phrase, he or she may not understand under which circumstances and context this phrase is to be used, and therefore, use it out of context. This falls under the category of incoherent speech.

Echolalia has resulted in disputes and debates among the scientific community. For scientists like *Uta Frith, Prizant* and others, echolalia is evidence of Gestalt processing. The term *Gestalt* belongs to the Berlin School of Psychology and indicates an attempt to separate, acquire and keep perceptions of meaning out of an apparently chaotic world.

On the other hand, *Tager-Flusberg* and *Calkins* conducted a study in 1990 on the acquisition of grammar by autistic children which showed that echolalia did not actually facilitate or contribute in any way to the grammatical development of people with AS.

Corresponding to echolalia, many aspies use **echopraxia**. Just like echolalia mimics sounds, echopraxia mimics body and hand motions and gestures. Both echolalia and echopraxia are imitated without explicit awareness of what actually is meant and why.

If these imitative behaviors are performed by aspies on their own they may mean nothing. But if they are conducted within the guidelines of behavioral therapies, they may have a very positive result. According to the stipulations of the study of *Ganos et al.* in 2012, both echolalia and echopraxia are useful, normal and necessary components for teaching social skills. As the study puts it:

"The imitating observer acquires new behaviors by reenacting previously shown motor or vocal patterns."

The distinction between actually learning and simply imitating cannot be made until the child reaches the age of three, when he or she starts to develop the ability to self-regulate.

It is rather evident from all the relevant studies that the problems of speech and language are derived from problems in perception. When the normal people use the word "window," they could mean "window of opportunity." The aspie does not comprehend this notion. When he or she uses the word "window," he or she means it literally.

On the other hand, this does not mean that all the people with AS have linguistic problems. On the contrary, it has been well documented that children with AS may have unusually sophisticated vocabularies and that their use of language is advanced for their ages.

This is where behavioral therapies focus. They teach the nuances and other meanings of words so that the aspie may acquire broader knowledge of language and, therefore, become able to better integrate socially.

Chapter 6: Effects of the Syndrome on Motor and Sensory Perception

The issue of physical clumsiness has been repeatedly mentioned in the previous chapters. It's time to elaborate on how Asperger's affects the motor and sensory perceptions of an individual.

The first thing to mention at this point is that motor and sensory perception problems may be independent of the diagnosis. They do affect the individual that suffers from the syndrome and their family, but they are not particularly sought out when the diagnosis is being made.

Motor perception is actually an improper term scientifically. The proper term is ***perceptual motor development*** and is defined as a person's ability to receive, understand and respond to information provided by the five senses of the human body. An aspie may have difficulty or inability in any of the three components of this definition. The clinical evidence so far indicates that the majority of aspies fail to understand what their minds are receiving, resulting in an inability to provide an appropriate response.

Sensory perception is the information received by a stimulus to any of the five senses of the body (touching, smelling, hearing, seeing, tasting) and the transmission of this information through the nervous system to the brain, where it will be processed by the motor perception. Clinical evidence shows that unless there is another medical condition in co-existence (myopia, reduced hearing, deaf-muteness, etc.), there are no significant problems in the way the senses work in people with AS.

Motor and sensory perception defects pertain to motor skills, sleep and emotions. Actually the term *defects* is incorrect, as aspies, in most cases, have such excellent visual and auditory perception that even the slightest of changes in a familiar environment is immediately noticed. Aspies' difficulties lie mostly in tasks that need a combination of visual and spatial perception and/or auditory and visual memory.

The auditory and visual memories especially present a problem. The term *memory* implies that something is stored in the brain to be accessed and used again at a later time. Visual memory of a fire, for example, recalls that if one gets too close to the flame, one will be burned. Auditory memory of an object maintains that if one scratches a specific object with a piece of metal, the resulting sound will be thoroughly unpleasant.

Aspies may be unusually perceptive to sound, light and other stimuli. On the other hand, they might also be totally insensitive to the exact same stimuli. The clinical evidence so far seems to be more in support of the hypothesis of decreased responsiveness to sensory input almost to the point of no reaction at all, even though there have been several recorded cases of exactly the opposite.

But no matter how acute their perception of sound and light may be, it does them no good if they cannot correlate an image or a sound with a situation. And that may be unnecessary if the sensation produced is positive or pleasant. But what happens if the sensation is negative? They are forced to relive the same unpleasant experience again and again unless there is an intervention.

A most worrying issue in the motor and sensory perception, directly linked to the problems of auditory and visual memory, is that there may not be any ***flight-or-fight*** mechanism. This is the mechanism that makes people respond to danger either by standing and fighting or by fleeing, and is one of the most vital physiological defensive mechanisms in humans.

Aspies may just stand there and do nothing at all when an attack or other harmful event occurs or when a threat to survival is present. This is one of the main reasons that they are subject to manipulation, victimization and bullying and that constant supervision is required.

The flight-or-fight mechanism depends upon discharges of the sympathetic nervous system. Hormones like estrogen and testosterone and neurotransmitters like dopamine and serotonin are released throughout the human body for the purpose of priming it to either fight or flee. If the danger is not correctly perceived then these substances will not be released and the body will be helpless and unable to respond.

To make matters worse, aspies are much more prone to ***habituation*** than others. Habituation is the condition when a person stops to respond to a situation after repeated exposure. A normal person may stop responding to a sound once he or she realizes that this sound is inconsequential and presents no adverse effects. The same stands true with an image or any other external stimulus.

A normal person may even bring himself or herself to not respond to a harmful stimulus after training and special precautions have been put into place. Unfortunately, when an aspie does not comprehend the harm that may come from a stimulus, he or she may reach habituation without any provisions, training or special precautions taken to avoid being hurt.

While what we have described so far are the most dire situations, the motor and sensory perception problems may be present in simpler, everyday functions and activities that a person suffering from AS may not be able to understand.

The problems in this aspect of the syndrome were first mentioned by Asperger himself. Riding a bicycle, opening a jar, and other functions requiring even the simplest of motor dexterities are acquired after a significant delay by children suffering from AS. At the same time, aspies may move awkwardly or, as Asperger put it, *"they do not feel comfortable in their own skins."*

Their hand-to-eye coordination is poor, their motion synchronization is poor, their posture may be odd or bouncy, their handwriting may even be unreadable and they may have problems with proprioception, which is the understanding of the body's position. They are also sometimes off-balance, and if they are asked to walk in tandem gait (with the toes of the back foot touching the heel of the front foot), they may not be able to.

The next problem in reference to motor skills and sensory perception is sleep. Children with Asperger's are prone to a bad quality of sleep, frequently waking up during the night or very early in the morning. They may also have difficulty in falling asleep altogether. It is not an unusual practice for the parents of a child with AS to induce sleep by giving him or her a mild sedative or valerian.

Relevant studies have shown that 73% of AS cases experience such problems and that there may be a unique physiological reaction involved. The evidence shows that the problems in motor and sensory perception may prevent these children from reaching REM, or rapid eye movement, sleep. During a normal REM phase, the release of neurotransmitters (namely serotonin) is completely halted. The result is an almost complete paralysis of the body due to motor neuron inhibition.

This entire sequence of events is actually absent in the sleep cycles of aspies. The result is known as REM behavior disorder. People in this state actually repeat the actions of from their dreams and experience parasomnias, which are transitional stages between wakefulness and non-REM sleep. This is why most AS children are more sluggish and disoriented when they wake up.

Poor sleep is bad for any medical situation. Good quality of sleep is a well-known remedy because it allows the body to heal itself. For the children with AS, the impact is unequivocal. It prompts negative mood swings, aggravates selective attention problems and further impairs cognitive functions.

Using sedatives to remedy the sleep problems is actually a bad idea, with the exception of chamomile. Parents need to get used to the notion that their children will resist sleep at first and then they will slowly grow accustomed to these changes. So far the most effective remedies in the case of AS are physical exercise, which will tire the body and force it to seek rest, alteration of the diet and changes in the bedroom environment and the sleep routine. Parents should also be aware that when they implement these changes, the sleeping situation may get worse before it improves.

In reference to physical exercise, apart from discharging the energy of the body, there is another objective involved. For about thirty to forty-five minutes before bedtime it is recommended that there should be a period of relaxation during which all sources of stimuli, like TV, radio, computer, Xbox or PlayStation and music, should be turned off. This will decrease the arousal of the child and help him or her to sleep better. For that matter, it is even recommended that parents remove all such sources from their child's bedroom.

The recommended diet alterations for people with AS involve avoidance of any foods containing high fat and MSG (monosodium glutamate), along with large meals two to three hours before bedtime. There should also be no use alcohol, tobacco or caffeine. Instead, food rich in proteins should be consumed along with a small carbohydrate/protein snack or milk before bedtime. For the children that wake up in the middle of the night to use the bathroom and then cannot fall asleep again, fluid consumption should be restricted in the two hours before going to bed.

On the subject of changing the sleep routine, the fact the aspies follow repetitive patterns may actually come in handy, as the best course of action is to set and maintain a specific hour of going to bed and waking up each morning. This routine should include the weekends, as many parents have the bad habit of allowing their children to sleep later and wake up later on a non-school day.

When a child wakes up late, it is difficult to go to sleep at the pre-arranged time. Keep in mind that it is much easier to wake up a sleeping child than putting an active child to sleep. If a child has trouble falling asleep and does not follow repetitive patterns, the following trick can be used when the change is implemented.

The first few nights the child is allowed to sleep whenever they feel tired but his wake up time must be kept the same. At some point, he will fall asleep ten minutes after he was put to bed. When this happens, the bedtime should be moved fifteen minutes earlier. This process is to be repeated until the desired bedtime is reached.

It is important for the child that the bedroom is not associated with activity but kept strictly as a sleeping environment. Temperature should be regulated to avoid extremes and, if possible, kept at the same level constantly. Light increases are associated with corresponding decreases in the release of melatonin, which in turn, triggers the child to wake up. Thus, it is important to make arrangements so that sunlight streams in the bedroom as early in the morning as possible.

Under the same premise and of equal importance is to darken the room at nightfall. In actuality, this is a suggestion that is not limited to children with AS but can be extended to all children who have trouble falling asleep. If the child displays fear of the dark, some psychotherapy may be required. And any clocks existing inside the bedroom should be removed. Watching the time may be a stressing factor causing anxiety.

These changes will require persistence and patience, but what the parents stand to provide for their children through regulating their sleep patterns and allowing them to get good-quality sleep is priceless. Their children will be in better moods when they wake up and in general, they will be capable of sustained attention and their overall health will be improve.

Unfortunately, there may be children suffering from AS of an extreme severity for which none of the above sleep remedies may be effective. If this is the case, a sleep expert should be contacted to provide guidance and advice or provide an appropriate solution. It could also be very useful to talk to other parents of children with AS who may have relevant experience.

Some people and cultures favor a siesta. This is highly inadvisable for children with AS especially if they have difficulty falling asleep. If they sleep during the day, it will be all the more difficult to get them to sleep again when it's time to go to bed at night.

The last major problem in sensory perception that we will examine is the one of *alexithymia*. The term defines the difficulty or inability to identify and describe the emotions of either oneself or others. The word is derived from the Greek word *αλεξιθυμία,* which literally means "no word for emotion."

In a most peculiar classification, alexithymia is considered as a personality trait. People displaying this conduct are considered to be at risk for developing medical and psychiatric conditions, and they may not respond to treatments that are administered through conventional means.

The exact medical definition includes:

➢ The difficulty of identifying emotions and distinguishing between an emotion and a bodily function that creates the emotion.
➢ The difficulty of describing their emotions to other people.
➢ Limited imagination.
➢ A cognitive style, which is extremely oriented and bound by stimuli.

The best description for aspies suffering from alexithymia is given by *Henry Krystal*:

"They think in an operative fashion and appear adjusted to reality more than expected. However, in psychotherapy, the cognitive deficiency becomes apparent as they tend to use monotonous detail, when recounting trivial actions and reactions in chronological order."

To be exact and accurate, it is not a total inability to express emotions that is included in alexithymia. Most often aspies will describe their emotions in single words like "sad" or "happy." But they cannot explain themselves any further than that. They may appear not to know what these emotional words mean.

Alexithymics feel emotional detachment from themselves, and, due to their inability to distinguish between emotions, they have considerable trouble in interpersonal relationships. This causes more severe medical problems like anxiety and depression and, in general, a lack of satisfaction in life. This is true even if the medical conditions are dealt with and controlled.

Under the pressure of all these factors put together, it is most common for alexithymics to discharge their frustration through completely impulsive and unconsidered actions, or through compulsive behaviors including substance abuse, anorexia nervosa and perverse sexual habits.

If no way is found to control and regulate these emotions, the end result will be a prolonged elevation of the autonomic nervous system, the neuroendocrine system and somatic diseases.

Chapter 7: Misunderstandings and Misjudgments of the Social Surroundings

In the previous chapters, we discussed how other people may perceive and understand their own interpersonal relationships with people suffering from Asperger Syndrome. It is now time to discuss and provide solutions to these various misunderstandings, misconceptions and misjudgments of society.

Tackling these issues in a chronological order, we need to begin with infancy and childhood. More advanced societies have no problem taking their children to a doctor for an examination if they suspect that there might be something wrong with their child. But less developed societies face a serious problem, that of social isolation.

The human species may have advanced away from the Spartan society (which murdered all the children that even looked like they were not strong enough to survive the Spartan lifestyle), but societies and religions still exist where any form of mental illness is treated with the incarceration to a lunatic asylum. Sufferers may be given some food and left there, unattended, until the end of his or her days.

Despite the efforts to educate and familiarize societies with the concept that not all mental disorders present a danger to society through violent and criminal behavior, there are still people that believe that any person suffering from such a disorder is a curse or an abomination and should be treated as such. For various reasons (most of them pertaining to fear, lack of knowledge, religion and distrust of doctor's opinions) many societies choose not to accept aspies within their ranks.

Let us repeat and **emphasize** these facts about people suffering from Asperger Syndrome:

A) Most often, they are the victims of manipulation, bullying and extortion. This, by definition, means that _under no circumstances do aspies present a danger to society and other people_. They may present a danger to themselves, but that's as far as it goes!

B) In the vast majority of cases, they do not even appear in public unless they have to. And, again, in most of their social appearances, either they are not noticed, or if they do, it's just by speaking in a monotonous tone or clinging to a single topic. How can this be considered dangerous to society?

C) If we cannot accept that they suffer from a disorder **and that it is not their fault that they do**, we cannot be considered empathetic humans ourselves. We do to them exactly what we accuse them of doing to us: being insensitive and disregarding of the feelings of other people.

Unfortunately, no matter what is said, religious fanaticism is a trait that will take a lot more than communication about medical conditions to change, and it is really a matter of serious debate why people do not trust doctors. To conclude on this point, people should not fear or be ashamed to take their children for an examination if they suspect that there might be something wrong. One of the most important aspects of proper treatment of the syndrome is that the correct diagnosis is made as early as possible.

And now we need to address another important and related issue, pride and scandal. It's time to discuss those parents who consider it a blow to their own pride that their children display the symptoms of Asperger's and those parents that think that if the world learns about their child's condition, it will create a scandal.

Parents are supposed to love their children no matter what. And they are expected to do everything to ensure their welfare and wellbeing. They must also do everything in their power to see to it that any medical problems that may appear during childhood are dealt with.

Many parents have been heard saying, or rather, shouting, "This child cannot be mine!" Why? Because he or she displays symptoms of a syndrome for which they are not even responsible? Because it might be the parents themselves that transferred the genetic heritage to their offspring? Because it was just bad luck that this condition happened?

No matter what the responses to these questions might be, it happened. Now what? Just leave them be? Lock them up some place that no one will ever learn of their existence? Is that human behavior? Is that human decency? And we use the term human and not parental. No matter what happened, parents **must be** parents, and do whatever it takes for their children to thrive.

They cannot let their pride or the fear of a scandal interfere with the timely diagnosis of the problem and the intervention that may be the key to a normal life for the child. It's not a matter of name, money and history; it's a matter of human dignity.

The second point to be made is school. Sometimes, aspies are more advanced than the rest of the children at school in the fields of mathematics, chemistry, biology or other classes. There have been many cases which document that people suffering from mental disorders are extremely adept and notice things that others miss.

For them, the subject matter which is taught in the classroom may be mundane and boring. Typical homework assignments may even be frustrating. This **does not mean** that the students are arrogant, spiteful or insubordinate, as some teachers consider them to be and punish them accordingly. It only means that some other method must be devised to maintain their interest in the field and help them advance further.

Punishment and chastising can only result in negative situations for aspies, and this may make some perfectly good individuals with great prospects withdraw and isolate themselves from society and never accomplish anything. If teachers cannot understand by themselves or be taught in seminars how they should handle aspies, then special schools may be in order. It is question worthy what would happen to Nobel Prize winner Vernon L. Smith, if his teachers did not recognize his potential for accomplishment.

It is even more worrisome how many other Vernon L. Smiths disappeared because their teachers, and the reactions they received at school in general, forced them to withdraw to solitude.

The biggest shortcoming is the lack of support and understanding for these people. _They are not evil, they are not dangerous and they are not devils._ They are just people suffering from a disorder that they did not cause themselves.

Most of the problems and the symptoms pertaining to the patients of the Asperger

Syndrome are limited to childhood and adolescence in more than 50% of cases. After adulthood, the problems may lessen or even disappear. Adult aspies actually have decided for themselves to do something about how society perceives them.

Some people view their opinions as extreme. Some others agree with them. Most others are indifferent. These opinions are presented in internet sites like *Wrong Planet*, while a subculture of aspies has been formed to allow them to communicate and exchange their views freely.

The main claim that aspies bring forth is that they should be recognized as different and not as people suffering from a disorder or a disability. For them, Asperger Syndrome is similar to homosexuality and people that display the symptoms should be treated and respected likewise. They claim that just like homosexuality was removed from the standard Diagnostic and Statistical Manual, so should Asperger's be removed.

To their cause, they have enlisted some very prominent figures, like that of the University of Cambridge Professor of Developmental

Psychopathology *Simon Baron-Cohen,* who is also a Fellow of Trinity College. His view on the subject as published in a paper in 2002, is:

"In society, there may be no great benefit by an eye with an ability for precise detail. But in mathematics, cataloging, music, computing, engineering and science in general, and eye for detail would probably lead to success, greatness and accomplishment rather than failure."

According to Baron-Cohen, there are only two reasons to keep the classification of aspies as a disorder or a disability. The first one is to maintain the provisions for the special support that is legally required, and the second is to recognize the emotional difficulties that result from the reduced empathy exhibited by aspies.

He concludes his views by mentioning that the genes behind Asperger's combination of abilities have existed throughout the human history and that they have made remarkable contributions to its evolution.

The concept behind the whole debate is that there neither is, nor ever should be, a brain configuration that is considered to be "ideal" and that normal people should comply with. Nor should any deviation from what is considered normal by considered as a pathology to be treated and remedied.

Just like the term *"neurotypical"* is used to describe people with normal neurological development, the term *"neurodiverse"* should be used to describe people with neurological developments that are considered to be deviating from the normal parameters.

It seems that there is a marked difference between adult aspies, who seem not to want to be changed and are actually proud of their diversity, and the parents who consider Asperger Syndrome a problematic situation that needs to be resolved at all costs (assuming that there are no pride and scandal issues involved).

No matter what the outcome of this debate might be at the level of legislature and regulation, the basis of the issue should be that it is neither a shame nor a curse if a child suffers from AS. At least this is what *Liane Holiday Willey* maintains in her books on the subject.

This is a story worth looking at. Liane Willey was born in 1959. She went through life and nobody noticed her abnormalities for **forty years!** She was diagnosed with Asperger's in 1999. And what did she do about it? She published:

➢ *"Pretending to be Normal"* in 1999

➢ *"Asperger Syndrome in the Family: Redefining Normal"* in 2001

➢ *"Adolescents and Asperger Syndrome in the Adolescent Years: Living with the Ups and Downs and Things in Between"* in 2003

➢ *"Safety Skills for Asperger Women: How to Save a Perfectly Good Female Life"* in 2011

She also founded the Asperger Society of Michigan.

If Willey fits the definition of evil, the devil or a danger, then these terms must be redefined and radically at that. However, it would probably be a lot easier to separate Siamese children than try to change centuries' long religious indoctrination and dogmatic view on what is or what is not normal.

Another despairing fact was shown in a study conducted in England in 2007. The general population may be aware of what autism and Asperger Syndrome are, but they have never been informed or educated about the experience of actually living with one. Similar studies were conducted in other countries with likewise results.

These studies indicate that there is a serious lack of publications which would inform the public of what needs to be done when they are faced with a situation where they must interact with an aspie. The vast majority of the available published works deal with the definitions and the nuances *but not usable advice or information about actions.*

These studies go one step further in mentioning that the general population has only been advised about autism and the autism spectrum and that very few people are actually aware that there is a marked difference between general autism and Asperger Syndrome. In fact, most people have not even heard the term.

What is even more frustrating for the aspies and their families is the conclusion of thesis studies. The vast majority of the general population responded, to the relevant questions, that they would be far more in favor and accepting of a person displaying the Asperger symptoms if they had previously been informed about it. If they were taught what they were supposed to do and how they would need to address aspies, they would be more comfortable and willing to modify their behaviors.

It is obvious that a systematic effort must be devised to educate the general population about Asperger's syndrome (and autism in general), not only as a condition or a disability but also as a form of living that requires some attention and some effort from those that society calls normal and science calls "neurotypical."

If this gets under way, the next time a person meets someone who speaks in a monotonous voice about a single topic and seems to not pay attention to attempts to change the topic, he or she may understand that they are not dealing with a person with a weird personality trait but an individual who may be suffering from the symptoms of Asperger's. And they may choose to adjust their behavior accordingly, instead of getting incensed.

Chapter 8: Therapies and Medication

For the time being and until the issues that we discussed in the previous chapters are resolved, Asperger Syndrome is considered as a disorder, and it's being managed by mainstream medicine through therapies and medication. The focus of the various treatments is to reduce the symptoms and to teach age-appropriate skills which may be missing from the patient.

As aforementioned, the therapies that may be used involve a multidisciplinary set of therapists and doctors in treatments that are prescribed on a case-by-case basis, as there is no single course of action which would cover the syndrome in general. Unfortunately, the data pertaining to how much progress has or has not been made is limited and it's inadvisable to extract any conclusions.

Medication

The nature of the syndrome, and the symptoms exhibited and pertaining to Asperger's itself, are not treatable by any medication. What needs medication and is treated accordingly is the existence of any comorbid conditions that, if left untreated, will result in more serious problems. This is but one more reason it is most imperative to diagnose the correct conditions as early as possible and why it is necessary for more than one doctor to get involved in the diagnostic process.

In many cases, the syndrome is accompanied with anxiety, depression, inattention and aggression. For these cases the atypical antipsychotics *risperidone* and *olanzapine* have displayed effectiveness in reducing the associated symptoms. Risperidone reduces the repetitive behavior which can induce self-injuries, can limit the outbursts of aggression and impulsiveness, and improve behaviors in social relationships and stereotypical patterns.

To improve on the restrictive and repetitive interests and behaviors, selective serotonin reuptake inhibitors (SSRIs) such as *fluvoxamine, fluoxetine* and *sertraline* have also proved effective.

There is one more issue to discuss in reference to medications. The occurrence of side effects is, in many cases, difficult to evaluate and may be dangerous. Patients of the autism spectrum are also routinely excluded from the tests and evaluations of the effectiveness of these medications against comorbid conditions.

Such side effects include an abnormal metabolism, an increased risk of type 2 diabetes, serious long-term neurological conditions and problems in cardiac conduction times. SSRIs may also have the opposite effect than the desired outcome regarding impulsiveness, aggression and sleep problems. Taking risperidone may result in weight gain and fatigue, which increase the risk of restlessness and dystonia. The use of sedatives may also have an impact in the learning process at school.

As amply displayed, medication, unless there are other conditions present, can be used only on certain occasions and to treat very specific situations. Otherwise, they may cause more problems than those they are called upon to solve. Treatment of AS relies heavily on the implementation of other cognitive therapies.

Therapies

For a total treatment of AS, many different therapies must be coordinated and focused together on addressing the core symptoms, such as the poor communication skills and the restrictive and repetitive routines. Linguistic capabilities, verbal strengths and deficiencies, and nonverbal inadequacies must also be taken under serious consideration.

The typical treatment program includes:

A) **Applied Behavioral Analysis**

ABA (previously known as *behavioral modification*) is a set of techniques implemented to systematically intervene and modify abnormal social behaviors. In the case of AS, the technique used is intended as *social skills training* and its purpose is to improve interpersonal interactions and any other skills pertaining to or interfering with communication between people.

The main concept behind the application of ABA to people with Asperger's is the hypothesis that there is absence of a ***theory of mind.*** In abbreviation, TOM. is the ability to understand that a person's brain works in a series of mental states such as beliefs, intents, desires, knowledge, pretensions, etc., and that other persons operate in the same mental states as well. These conditions of the mind are different from person to person and the focus of the therapy is to make one person understand and accept his or her own mental states as well as those of others.

In this regard, children displaying Asperger's are a bit luckier than children displaying the symptoms of the other disorders of the autism spectrum, as their initial understanding of a social theory of mind is considerably higher.

The therapy focuses on theory of mind tasks. The concept is that the abilities involved in mental processes are subserved by a series of dedicated mechanisms. It is believed that these mechanisms are actually affected by the impairment, and not the cognitive functions themselves.

By assigning the TOM tasks, the hypothesis is that these dedicated mechanisms, which may otherwise be inactive, are put to work and serve their purposes, which is to support the overlaying cognitive functions. Consequently, the cognitive functions allow the individual to first comprehend about his or her own states of mind and then to understand how these mental states translate from one person to another.

B) **Cognitive Behavioral Therapy**

This is a common therapeutic tactic in all disorders that have to do with the brain. The objective is to improve *stress management* in reference to anxiety, depression and the emotions that produce explosive outbursts. The intervention also aims to reduce the obsessive occupation with interests and the constant repetition of the daily routines.

The objective of CBT is to improve everyday functioning. To achieve that goal it uses a number of techniques and physiotherapies. These fall under two major models.

The **transactional model** considers the stress as an imbalance between the demands made to one person and the resources this person has at his disposal to satisfy the demands. The problem occurs when the applied pressure on a person exceeds his or her ability to cope with the situation. The model focuses on this ability to cope with the problem and intervenes so that the stressing factor can be considered as a positive or even challenging notion instead of a threat.

The **health realization (or innate health) model** focuses on the thought processes, which determine the appropriate response to what is perceived as a potentially stressful situation.

In both models, there are over thirty techniques available, oriented to allow the person undergoing therapy to better manage his or her stress. A brief list of the techniques which are most used in AS therapies, looks like:

- ➢ Autogenic training
- ➢ Conflict resolution
- ➢ Cranial release
- ➢ Social activity
- ➢ Mindfulness
- ➢ Nootropics
- ➢ Artistic expression
- ➢ Somatics training
- ➢ Time management
- ➢ Planning and decision making
- ➢ Pets

C) **Occupational or Physical Therapy**

If any person anywhere and at any time finds any doctor of any discipline that will ever say that physical exercise is not a good thing, it should be a surprise of great magnitude. In the case of AS, these therapies aim at improving the sensory perception and the motor coordination abilities that are woefully absent, and are important in improving the psychological conditions rather than the physical ones.

One of the symptoms exhibited by aspies is physical clumsiness. **Sensory processing** is the sequence of events in the neurological system that interprets the input from the environment through the sensors of the body, and allows it to be used and interpreted in the most effective way.

The therapy intends to teach an aspie how to use his or her brain to process the modality input from multiple sources and understand concepts like:

a) **Proprioception**

This is the understanding of the relative position of the various parts of the body and the amount of effort required for movement.

b) **Tactile**

This is the understanding of the various sensations and emotions caused by the touch of the human body receptors to thermal, chemical, mechanical and light sources.

c) Olfactory
Similar to tactile, this has to do with the input provided by various odors and smells.

d) Vestibular system
This is the system in the body that is responsible for balance and spatial orientation. (Remember that aspies may not be able to walk in a tandem gait.)

e) Interoception
This is the normal and physiological capacity of any living organism to receive information and convert them to perception and then action or reaction and, consequently, be able to convert them to usable functions.

Motor coordination is the physical process that allows the human body to receive the inputs from kinematic and kinetic parameters and to form an intended action. A kinematic parameter references the spatial direction and a kinetic parameter references the amount of force required to move towards a certain point. A similar combination of parameters is the visual input from a moving object and the range of motion to be carried by the hand, which will allow it to capture the object that the eye is watching.

To put it simply, motor coordination is the process that allows the mind to order the body to make a motion, based on the input it receives through the five senses.

Aspies have problems in the neural process of the cerebellum which do not allow them to interpret the sensory input and, therefore, to order the body to take action. The therapy focuses on instructing the brain how to correctly perceive the input and then how to react accordingly.

D) **Speech Therapy**
We have repeatedly mentioned the way aspies speak. Specialized speech therapy is aimed at acquainting the aspie with the pragmatics of give-and-take during a normal conversation so that they no longer disregard or misinterpret the stance of the person to whom they are talking.

The therapy is to be administered by a speech-language pathologist. While the therapy should primarily focus on the pragmatics, lesser issues may involve therapy in:

a) **Phonation**

This is the sound production in the larynx. We have already discussed that when aspies talk, their voice may sound in a way that alienates the listener.

b) **Resonance**

The pitch of a voice is a matter of resonance. Aspies may talk without pitch. This part is aimed to introduce the importance of pitch in a voice pattern.

c) **Fluency**

When an aspie talks, he may sound incoherent. This part of the therapy is intended to match words with meanings.

d) **Intonation**

The monotonous style of speech is addressed in this part of the therapy.

e) **Pitch variance**

Pitch is an emotion indicator. Each pitch is associated with a different emotion.

f) **Morphology**

This is the part of the therapy which teaches how to speak in small sentences which make sense, using grammar and syntax rules.

To return to the pragmatics aspect of the therapy, this is the central part, as it teaches the ways by which context is transformed to meaning. Remember that sometimes, people suffering from the syndrome do not understand the meanings of what they are actually saying. Also, they do not have a grasp of sarcastic speech, metaphors, humor and other forms of conversational implicature.

These pragmatics are actually what teaches all people to speak in a way so that others can understand what they are saying and react to it.

E) **Positive behavior support**

This part of the therapy is not aimed at the patient. It is aimed at the families and the faculties at school, and its objective is to introduce behavioral management strategies to be used at home or school to support and tolerate the behavioral problems of an aspie.

The basic notion behind the training is to understand what lies behind and maintains the abnormal behavior. These behaviors serve a purpose for the aspies; they are functional. Children do not have to be suffering from the syndrome to display a certain behavior in the presence of adults in order to receive more attention and/or rewards.

The key is *functional behavior assessment*. It describes behaviors, marks the context in reference to time, events and circumstances, and predicts when the abnormal behavior will occur or not. The training involves:

a) **Identification of Goals**

   This is a two-prong effort. The first leg is to identify if the strategy selected is feasible in reference to the individual it will be implemented with, desirable by the individual (it will do no good if the patient resents it), and effective in obtaining the second leg, which is the specific behavioral adjustments that are needed.

b) **Gathering of Information**

An integral part of the effectiveness of any strategy is the correct observation of the behaviors at home and at school in association with the context issues. Behavioral patterns in aspies are repetitive, which means that there may be a certain time during the day that the abnormal behavior occurs. Or, a child displaying the symptoms may be perfectly normal until a derogatory comment or a bad joke is made, and then he or she becomes insulted and acts without thinking. Additionally, a class in school may be considered too mundane and boring for an aspie, and a different set of curricular activities may have to be devised to match his skills in a specific field.

All the above is necessary information so that the model of positive behavioral support implemented will produce the optimal effect.

c) **Development of a Working Hypothesis**
The first two of these steps yield the appropriate information, which, under

examination by an appropriate team of professionals, will determine the specific issues pertaining to the individual aspie who will undergo these strategic changes. There is a marked difference in the underlying dysfunctionality between an aspie who is focused and orderly and an aspie who cannot focus on anything and is completely disorderly.

d) **Designing a Support Plan**

After all the above steps have been completed, it is time to decide on what to do. How can a behavior occurring only at a specific time of the day be handled in a focused and orderly child? How can he or she handle a bad joke or a derogatory comment when he or she is completely impulsive?

This, and the implementation step, are actually the most important ones in the positive support training. If the wrong plan is devised, then no matter how well it is implemented, it is the wrong plan. It will yield no positive results.

e) **Implementation**

Once parents and teachers know what to do, they need to actually do it. They need to do it properly and most of all *willingly*. An aspie will sense if the instructions and the behavior of the parent or the teacher is forced, or resentful, or performed without their hearts in it. They will disregard the strategy altogether.

Assuming that the correct plan has been devised, both parents and teachers **must,** first of all, **be convinced** that it will provide the desired results. Then they **must project** the feeling that they will do whatever it takes **gladly** and **wholeheartedly**.

The implementation involves one last element which is the trickiest of them all: **patience.** If parents and teachers expect results immediately, they will be completely and utterly disappointed. Part of the training is to make them understand that it will not only take time to see improvements, but it may also be that despite their efforts, their child may show very little to no improvement at all, if the case is severe enough.

This part is especially tricky because many people are inherently impatient. They must first achieve this virtue themselves before being allowed to implement any strategy for positive behavior support on another individual.

f) **Monitoring**

The last issue of the training is to monitor the progress. This step will identify if the devised plan and its implementation were effective. If not, a revision may be required or the strategy may be altered altogether. Otherwise, just some tweaking may be required to some aspects of the strategy.

Therapies do not work on auto-pilot. There might be unintentional side-effects. These must be identified in the monitoring process and dealt with appropriately. And the most integral part of this process is that the parent and the teacher must always be in constant and immediate contact with the appropriate professionals who can guide and advise them in a proper and timely manner.

It is curious and noteworthy that the majority of the studies conducted on programs of early intervention that are behavior based are merely simple case reports of up to five participants. In most instances, they examine only a few problematic behaviors such as self-inflicted injuries, aggression, refusal to comply, spontaneous language and stereotypes, and completely ignore the existence of unintentional side-effects.

Other issues may have surfaced during the implementation of these therapies that were completely unexpected and, thus far, unexplained. For example, in a controlled study of the positive behavior support, a group of parents were trained in a one day workshop, while another group attended six individual lessons. The parents that attended the workshop reported *fewer* behavioral problems, while the parents that attended the individual lessons, reported *less intense* behavioral problems.

Such issues only reinforce the notion that there can be no single therapy for Asperger Syndrome, not only because aspies are very different from individual to individual, but also because those who are providing support, tolerance and understanding have a different level of comprehension of the nuances involved and a different attitude towards the implementation of the therapies.

As long as the core causes of the syndrome are not identified and medically or genetically dealt with, this will probably be the case, unless something really dramatic happens. Each individual case of a person that displays the symptoms of Asperger's will have to be treated differently and according to the specifics and the circumstances surrounding the specific individual.

Chapter 9: Alternative Therapies

Mainstream medicine and medical science is based on healing through evidence acquired by the scientific method, i.e. the observation, the measurement, the experimentation, the formulation of a hypothesis and the proof of the theory. Whenever this method fails to provide a solution to a certain medical problem for any reason, people turn to alternative methods of healing.

Alternative does not necessarily mean dangerous. In fact, alternative medicine is quite acceptable by the medical world. The only difference is that it is a set of methods intended to provide healing through empirical practices, secrets transferred between knowledgeable people, and ancient healing philosophies, such as the ones from China, which have not been tested yet by the relevant research as to their effectiveness. This only means that they have not followed the rule of evidence as acquired through the scientific method.

Alternative medicine employs a wide range of practices like homeopathy, naturopathy, energy medicine, acupuncture, Ayurvedic medicine, all the way to simple faith healing. For some of these practices, there is little evidence as to their effectiveness, but for some others there is more. And for many there is evidence of contradiction or interference with mainstream medicine in the same way as there is evidence acting in support or assistance to mainstream medicine.

At this point, and before the discussion on alternative ways to treat Asperger Syndrome begins, we would like to **strongly** recommend that before any decision is made to follow courses of action indicated by alternative ways, one should discuss these ways thoroughly with an appropriately trained professional who is the only person qualified to provide proper guidance and advice. Should there be a case where medications have been prescribed, there is evidence that some alternative practices interfere with their effectiveness and reduce it or negate it altogether.

There might also be evidence that, while one practice may provide a little effect, a combination of mainstream and alternative ways may provide a better effect. It is of the utmost importance that *no experimentation* should be decided upon on to treat AS without professional approval. The effects may be completely adverse, if not plainly catastrophic.

In the case of Asperger's, alternative ways of remedying the condition include:

A) **Intervention on the Dietary Habits**
Some categories of foods have been found to work effectively on certain areas of the brain and assist in the brain functions that have been impaired by the syndrome.

a) **Omega-3**
Omega-3 fat has been found to assist in the lining of the neural passageways. This allows the brain to acquire better communication with the body and decrease the behavioral issues faced by aspies. The brain function may be improved altogether.

Natural sources of omega-3 fatty acids are:

Flax

Hemp

Swordfish

Sardines

Pollock

Salmon

Halibut

Tuna

Herring

Greenshell

Tilefish

Mackerel

Broccoli

Cod

Flounder

Turkey

Red snapper

Gemfish

Catfish

Eggs

Lean red meat

Grouper

Cereals

Fruit

Milk

Apart from the effectiveness of omega-3, advice should be taken on the daily levels permitted per case. Due to environmental pollution, too much consumption of foods containing omega-3 may result in *heavy metal poisoning* from mercury, nickel, lead, arsenic and cadmium found in fish.

b) **Vitamin B6**

Food rich in B6 (otherwise known as pyridoxine) assists in the regulation of agitation, aggressiveness, depression and irritability. B6 improves the auditory-visual and auditory-tactile coordination, thus improving motor skill deficiencies. The greatest sources of B6 in nature are:

Sunflower seeds

Pistachio nuts

Tuna

Lean pork

Turkey

Dried fruit

Chicken

Lean beef

Bananas

Spinach

Avocado

Consumption of B6 above the recommended daily input for prolonged periods of time may be toxic and result in irreversible neurological conditions.

c) **Vitamin C**

Commonly known as niacin or nicotinic acid (no correlation with cigarettes or tobacco smoking), this is a powerful antioxidant used in conjunction with other vitamins. The effect on the brain is to reduce depressive symptoms, improve on the general brain function and assist in better regulation of behavioral issues. The food sources that should be included in the dietary habits are:

Liver, heart and kidneys

Chicken

Beef

Eggs

Tuna, salmon, halibut

Venison

Dates

Avocados

Leaf vegetables

Tomatoes

Broccoli

Carrots

Sweet potatoes

Asparagus

Nuts

Legumes

Whole grain products

Beer

Ovaltine

Peanut butter

Consumption should never exceed the recommended daily input. The side-effects include skin flushing, itching, dry skin, eczema exacerbation and acanthosis nigricans (brown or black velvety hyperpigmentation of the skin).

d) **Coconut oil**

Its concentration of capryllic acid helps in memory retention (as aforementioned there have been cases were the skill development was initially normal and then suddenly the skills were lost) and reduces the possibility of cognitive decline.

e) **Asian ginseng and green cardamom**

Both foods are strong antioxidants with neuro-protective properties, reducing aggressive and impulsive behaviors.

f) **Gingko Biloba**

It is an extract from the ginkgo tree that has displayed properties of improved brain circulation and memory retention.

g) **St. John's Wort**

This is an herb that has proven effective in reducing the levels of excitement and tension along with anxiety, fear and depression. It is also a very good mood enhancer.

h) **Chamomile**

Chamomile is a renowned natural sedative that can be used by those who display symptoms and suffer from sleep problems.

B) **Acupuncture**

Acupuncture and acupressure are linked to the neurology of the body. The practitioners claim that the application to the nerves accesses areas of the brain and change its functioning.

For an effective implementation on aspies, they must also be subjected to kinesiology treatment, nutritional interventions, a teaching of the basics of reflexology and recognition of sound and discrimination of color therapies.

The main problem the practitioners face when treating aspies is to persuade them to follow directions and to lay still (except when they are treated with scalp acupuncture).

C) **Ayurveda**

Kerala Ayurveda deals with all four types of autism. It deals with the disorders using a complete therapy which includes powder, pills and liquids, oil for massage and special care taken for the blood pressure, the digestion problems and the urine system of the persons under the treatment.

For reasons of better implementation and the achievement of more positive results, most of the practitioners require a full medical record accompanied with lab reports. All the medical compounds used are not offered for commercial usage and are specially manufactured on a per case basis.

Apart from the compounds, the basic teaching of ayuervedic medicine in reference to Asperger's, is ***pranayama*** which, loosely translated, means the "*extension of one's life force.*" Through fifty different techniques, it focuses on breathing and its effects on stress, autonomic functions and asthma.

Its practitioners maintain that pranayama helps greatly to develop a steady mind, a strong willpower and a judgment that is sound.

D) **Chinese Medicine**

Chinese medicine has been around for thousands of years just like Ayurveda. Although it has not been sufficiently researched by the Western scientific method, there is plenty of evidence that it is effective against a wide range of mental disorders through the use of herbs and botanicals that mainstream medicine knows very little about.

The main difference between Western and Chinese medicine is that Westerners consider the mind as the cornerstone of the human physique, while the Chinese consider the combination of mind and body as a single, undivided entity. For the Westerners, the emotional influence is a secondary effect on the organs of the body, while for the Chinese, it is the key that binds everything together and achieves balance.

The two main aspects that are strongly affected by all kinds of autism are *reason* and *awareness*. In Chinese medicine, these are controlled by the heart, the spleen and the kidney. The heart rules the mental functions including short-term memory and emotional states. The spleen regulates the mind's ability to concentrate, study and memorize. The kidney is responsible for long-term memory. Autism is any disturbance in the balance between these three areas.

The suggested remedies include eliminating phlegm, tonifying the blood of the heart, clearing the heat of the heart, and tonifying the essences of the spleen and the kidney.

The theory behind these remedies is that the existence of phlegm causes dull wits, speech that is incoherent, confusion in the mind, lethargy and limited attention to the environment. Phlegm is addressed as *phlegm fire* and is presented as: disturbed sleep harassing the heart, making people talk to themselves, causing emotional outbursts like laughing and crying that are uncontrollable, and inducing aggression, constipation and a short temper.

The *spleen fire* and the *kidney fire*, if deficient, cause food intake problems (in the former instance) and poor mental development (in the latter instance). The *heart fire* deficiencies will cause lethargy, fidgety restlessness and/or aggressive behavior.

Key to the successful remedies is a dietary reform. A good diet should avoid yeast, casein, glutens and any allergens, and focus on flavor (salty, sweet and pungent), temperature and affects on the body. The food must be warm and not extreme.

The Chinese claim that such remedies have been successful for 5,000 years. The Western world has decided not to put them to any effect until they are fully researched. Unfortunately, any such study takes an inordinate amount of time, and nothing has been proven yet.

At this time, resorting to the Chinese methods is a question of trust in the Chinese tradition, history and knowledge. It may be helpful or appealing for those that do not trust Western doctors.

Both medical styles (mainstream and alternative) strive to heal. It is not a question of which one is right or wrong or more effective. It's possible that they both are right and wrong, effective and ineffective, all at the same time. Or it may be that a combination of both can provide the optimal results.

Chapter 10: Medical Conditions That Maybe Present At the Same Time as Asperger Syndrome

As already mentioned, there are cases where people with AS also suffer from co-existing medical conditions. Some of them are mental, but some of them are not. Co-existing medical conditions that have been recorded to accompany Asperger's and do not affect a differential diagnosis are:

A) **Tuberous Sclerosis**

This is a rare genetic disorder that works in multiple systems and produces benign tumors in the brain and other vital organs like the kidneys, the heart, the lungs and the skin. It is caused by mutations of the genes TSC1 and TSC2, which are responsible for the coding of the proteins *hamartin* and *tuberin,* and it has a consistently strong association with AS. 1 to 4% of individuals with Asperger's also have this disorder.

B) **Sensory Problems**

When the perceptions of children are accurate, they can learn from their visual, auditory and feeling input. On the other hand, if the sensory input is abnormal, the children's experiences about the world can be confusing.

Many children with AS are highly attuned or oversensitive (sometimes painfully) to certain sounds, tastes, textures, images and smells. Some children consider the feeling of clothes touching their skin almost intolerable. Some auditory inputs such as a vacuum cleaner, a sudden storm, a ringing phone, or even the sound of waves lapping at a shore may force these children to cover their ears or eyes and scream.

In AS, as aforementioned, the brain seems unable to regulate and balance the senses. Some children with AS can be oblivious to extreme cold, heat or pain. Such a child may fall and break a bone and yet never cry. Another may hit his or her head against a wall and not even flinch, but it is also possible that a light touch may make the same child scream in agony.

C) **Seizures**

25% of children with AS develop seizures, often starting either in early childhood or during adolescence. These seizures are caused by abnormal electrical activity in the brain and can produce a temporary loss of consciousness (regularly referred to as a "blackout"), a convulsion in the body, staring spells or unusual movements. A contributing factor to these seizures may be lack of sleep or a high fever.

An EEG (electroencephalogram, an examination that records the electric currents developed in the brain by attaching electrodes to the scalp) can confirm the presence of a seizure.

In most cases, seizures can be controlled by medical compounds called "anticonvulsants." The dosage needs to be regulated carefully so that the least possible quantity of medication may be used for effectiveness.

D) **Mental Retardation**
Many kids with Asperger syndrome have mental impairment of various levels of severity. When they are examined, some of their abilities may be normal, while some

others may be particularly weak. For example, a child with AS may do well on the parts of the test that evaluate visual skills but score poorly on the language tests.

E) **Fragile X Syndrome**
This is the most commonly inherited kind of mental retardation. It earned the name due to the fact that one part of the X chromosome (X being the part that represents the father) has a defective component that appears pinched and fragile when placed under a microscope.

The syndrome affects about 2 to 5% of aspies. It is important to have a child with AS examined for Fragile X Syndrome, especially if the mothers and fathers are considering having another child. For some inexplicable reason, if a child suffers from both syndromes, there is a 50% chance that boys born to the same parents will have the syndrome as well. In this case, it is advisable for other members of the family, who may be considering having a child, to undergo an examination for the syndrome.

There is no distinction between a father's and a mother's ability to pass along the altered gene to their offspring. As both males and females have at least one X chromosome, they can both can pass the mutated gene on to their children. But there is a distinction to be made.

A father will only pass the altered gene on to his daughters. The sons get a Y chromosome, which doesn't transmit the syndrome. Should the father have the altered gene, but the mother's chromosomes are normal, all of the couple's daughters will have the altered gene, but none of their sons.

Mothers pass only the X chromosomes on to their children. If it is the mother who has the altered gene for Fragile X, she can pass it on to all of her children regardless if the father has it or not. The only thing that changes is the chances of inheriting the syndrome, which vary from 50% to 100% (if the father has the defective gene as well).

The latest statistics show that 5% of individuals with autism or Asperger's also have the Fragile X Syndrome, while 10% to 15% of those with Fragile X have autistic or Asperger's traits.

Sometimes, with the tests to determine if a child falls under the qualifications of Asperger Syndrome, it is advisable to ask for additional tests to determine if there are other, co-existing conditions. Otherwise treating AS without taking the other conditions into consideration may have no effect.

Chapter 11: Available Aids

When a child has been examined and diagnosed with AS, the parents may feel ill-equipped to help their child develop to the full extent of his or her abilities. As they begin to look at the available options for treatment, they should also look for available types of aid for a child with a disability. They will find out that there is plenty of help available that they can use.

It is not going to be easy to learn and memorize everything needed to know about the resources that will provide the greatest assistance. It is advisable for parents to write everything down and to keep the notes handy when they need to recall appropriate information.

They should also keep a record of the physicians' reports and the evaluations that their child has been given, so that his or her eligibility for special programs is thoroughly documented.

The next step is to look for and learn everything they can about any special programs that may be available for their child; the more they know, the more effectively they can advocate and make sure that their child is receiving all the help he or she can get.

For every child that is deemed eligible for a special program, each state guarantees the existence of special education and all the related services. The Individuals with Disabilities Education Act (IDEA) is a program federally directed that ascertains free and appropriate public education for children with learning deficits after they are diagnosed and certified as such.

Usually, the children are allocated to public schools, and all the necessary services, such as a speech therapist, an occupational therapist, a school psychologist, a social worker or a school nurse on an as-needed basis, are paid for by the school district.

According to the relevant legislature, the public schools must prepare and perform a set of instruction objectives, or specific skills, for every child that has been enrolled in a special education program.

The list of skills is known as the children's Individualized Education Program (IEP). An IEP is actually an agreement between the family and the school on the child's objectives. When a child's IEP is developed, the family will be asked to attend a meeting. At this meeting, there will be several individuals present, including a special education teacher, a representative of the public schools who has the necessary knowledge about the program, and other individuals invited by the school or by the family (relatives, a child care provider, or a close friend who knows the child well and is supportive).

Mothers and fathers also play an important part in the creation of the program, as they know their child and his needs best. Once a child's IEP is developed and is underway, a meeting is scheduled once a year to review the child's progress and to make any adjustments necessary to accommodate his or her changing needs.

If a child is under the age of three and has certified special needs, he or she should be eligible for an early intervention program which is also available in every state.

Each state appoints a specific agency as the lead one in this early intervention program. The services of this program are provided by workers eminently qualified to care for children with disabilities and usually come to the child's home or another place that is familiar to the child.

The services to be provided are agreed upon into an Individualized Family Service Plan (IFSP) that is reviewed at least once in every 6 months. The plan will precisely describe the services that will be provided to the child, but it will also describe the services for the parents, which are intended to assist them with the daily activities that involve their child, and for any siblings to adjust to having a brother or sister with Asperger's at home.

Chapter 12: Advice on What to do in Various Encounters with People Suffering from Asperger Syndrome

Most of the time, people do not know how to handle and how to treat a person with AS. As shown in the relevant research discussed above, this is one of the problems that results from the social interaction problems between aspies and the general population.

Asking for help is never a problem and such help concerns both the people who are related to the person with Asperger's and people that may come in contact with an aspie in a social occasion. Here are some of the issues that need to be addressed.

A child has been rejected, mocked and bullied by his classmates.

This is a usual complaint made by parents of children with AS. Social rejection results in devastating effects in an aspie's social functioning. Because they tend to internalize how others treat them, any possible rejection will damage their self-esteem and, in many cases, it will cause anxiety and depression.

As the child comes to feel worse about themselves and anxiety and depression set in, they perform worse both socially and intellectually. This is the main aspect focused on by the social skill training techniques as discussed in Chapter 8.

Unfortunately, many children and teens with AS have never been taught such interpersonal skills as "small talk" in social settings, the importance of good eye contact during a conversation, or knowing when to speak and when to listen, etc.

If this issue is not properly addressed by an appropriate specialist, as the years go by, the child with AS will rapidly become reduced to a person who is surviving on:

- Anger, hate and resentment towards other people
- Feeling that he or she is a mistake
- Isolation
- Low self-esteem and self-hate
- Sadness

If this truly is the case, then alarm bells should be going off and changes are urgently required.

Furthermore, many of these children have never learned how to interpret the many subtle cues contained in social interactions. This is also an issue to be addressed at social skills training.

The training assumes that when children improve on their social skills or change some of their behaviors, their self-esteem will increase considerably, along with the possibilities that others will respond favorably to them.

To achieve all the above, a parent **must** have his child practice selected behaviors again and again until they become something of a second nature. They also need to disregard any resentment displayed by their child in this process but **NOT forcibly.** They need to override the child's objection in a way so that they know he or she will finally accept the teachings.

How to Prevent Meltdowns

Meltdowns are usual in people with AS and are not a pretty sight. They are something like exaggerated temper tantrums, only meltdowns can last from a few minutes to well over an hour.

When a meltdown starts, the child is completely out-of-control. When it ends, both the parents and the child are completely exhausted. But... it's not over yet. At the slightest of provocations, for the remainder of the day (sometimes into the next one as well) the meltdown can come back in full force.

It should be expected that children with AS will experience both major and minor meltdowns over events that are part of daily life. They may have a major meltdown over a very small event, or a minor one over something that is or can be considered as a major issue. There is no way to tell how they are going to react when they are faced with certain situations. However, there are many ways to help a child learn to control emotions.

It is a bad choice for a parent of an out of control child with AS to try to regain control. It will have little or no success no matter how hard they try. And it seems that the harder the parents try, the more out of control the child becomes.

The following statement often comes from parents:

"I have tried everything with him (or her)! Nothing works!"

This could not be further from the truth. They may, indeed, have tried, but they couldn't possibly have tried everything and or have tried to do it efficiently.

Just like their children, parents need training too. Some of the strategies that exist have an effect immediately, while some others produce results over a period of time.

Meltdowns are prevented by observation and identification. When a child goes into a meltdown for the same reason every time, then eliminating the reason prevents the meltdown. This is the immediate solution that provides results.

The long-term solution is to teach the child **at the child's own pace of learning** what emotions are and how to handle them. This teaching should only involve **one emotion at a time**.

This is the only durable solution that will prevent the meltdowns altogether. And never try to regain control when a meltdown occurs. Just be there to prevent any physical harm to come to your child. **Do not shout and do not react in anger.**

Parenting Defiant Teens with AS

Asperger's is at the less aggressive end of the autism spectrum. Nevertheless, the challenges parents face when disciplining a teenager with AS are much harder than with an average teen.

Complicated by defiant behavior, the teenager with AS is at risk of even greater difficulties on multiple levels, unless the parents' disciplinary techniques are formulated to take into account their child's special needs.

Parents need to devise a consistent disciplinary plan well ahead of time, and then present a unified front towards the offense that needs disciplining and continuously review their strategies for possible changes and improvements as their teenager develops and matures.

Parents must learn how to:

➢ Identity the concerning behavioral patterns
➢ Come to an agreement with their teenager on the "Asperger-specific" disciplinary actions to be taken

➢ Clearly post the rules and consequences included in this agreement

➢ Implement a system of rewards when the teenager complies with rules

➢ Not refrain from the application of the consequences tailored to the specific needs of the teenager

The behavioral and social deficiencies involved in Asperger's have already been discussed in detail. Due to these deficiencies, many teenagers may also experience the following associated problems:

A) Criminal Activity

Loneliness, despair and pain can lead to problems with controlled substances. In their overwhelming need to fit in and make friends, some teenagers hang out with the wrong high school crowds. "Average" teens who abuse substances may use the teenager's naivety to get them to buy or carry drugs and alcohol for their group.

Should they be cornered by a police officer, these teens usually do not have the skill to answer the officer's questions. In most cases, they will probably provide an answer that will get them in further trouble with the law.

B) Acting Out

The years of being a teenager are the more emotional for everyone. Yet the hormonal changes of adolescence combined with the deficiencies we've discussed may result in a teenager with AS becoming emotionally overwhelmed.

The tantrums and meltdowns may reappear. Boys often respond by physically attacking a teacher or a classmate. These meltdowns may be experienced at home after another day filled with irritation, bullying, pressure to adapt, and rejection in the end.

Suicide and addiction to drugs become real concerns, as the teenager now has access to means that can actually cause him- or herself physical harm. This period can overwhelm both a teenager with AS and their family.

C) Inability to act like other teenagers

A teen with AS typically does not care about fashions and clothing styles or any of the other concerns that obsess the other teens in their peer group. They may even neglect their hygiene and wear the same haircut for years. Boys forget or do not care about shaving; girls don't fix their hair or follow the current fashion in appearance.

Some teens remain stuck in the clothes they wore in grammar school and hobbies like unicorns and Legos, instead of moving into concerns like Facebook and dating with members of the opposite sex.

Some of the boys often have no motor coordination which leaves them out of high school sports, which, in turn, is a typically essential area of male bonding and friendship.

D) School Failures

Many teens with AS have average to above average IQs can sail through grammar school but face academic problems in middle and high school classes. They now have to deal with several teachers, instead of just the one they did before.

The probability that at least one of these teachers will be indifferent or even hostile towards making any special accommodations is a certainty. The teenager now has to face a series of classroom surroundings with different classmates, smells, distractions, noise levels, and, most of all, different sets of expectations.

The distractibility and difficulty to organize materials places a teen with AS in similar academic problems as students suffering from Attention Deficit Disorder. A term paper or a science project becomes impossible to manage because no one has taught them how to divide it up into a series of small steps.

Even though the academic stress can be overwhelming, school administrators may be reluctant to enroll teens with AS in a special education program at this late point in their educational careers.

E) Sexual Issues

Teens with AS are not aware of the "street knowledge" of sex and dating behaviors that other teens pick up normally. They are naive and clueless about sex and its notions.

Boys can face this problem by becoming preoccupied with internet pornography and masturbation. They can be exceedingly forward with a girl who may merely be kind, and then face charges of stalking her.

A girl may have a female body that is fully-developed and yet absolutely no understanding of romance and non-verbal sexual cues. This makes her vulnerable to sexual harassment, and she could wind up the victim in the event of teenage date rape.

F) Social Isolation

This is completely different than the social isolation issues already discussed.

Everyone feels insecure in the teenage world, and teens that appear different are often ostracized. Teens with AS often display odd mannerisms. Some may talk in a loud unchanging voice, may avoid eye contact, may interrupt others, may violate others' physical space, and may steer the conversation to their favorite topic.

Another may appear willful, selfish and remote, mostly because they are unable to share their thoughts and feelings with others. Isolated and alone, many teenagers with AS are too anxious to initiate social contact. Many of them are also rigid and rule-oriented and act like little adults, which is considered as a deadly trait in any popularity contest.

Friendship and all its nuances of reciprocity can be exhausting for an aspie, even though he or she wants it more than anything else. There have been recorded cases of teenagers with AS ending a close friendship with this statement:

"Your expectations are killing me. The telephone calls, the endless talks, all that you feel... it's just too much for me. I can't take it anymore."

Again, it is a matter of teaching a son or a daughter the rules, just like during childhood. But parents will have to make their son or daughter realize that they are no longer children and have advanced to the next level. If what works in this instance is to approach it like a game, wherein the player has advanced to the next level where new challengers will be faced, so be it!

Living with an Spouse or a Partner with Asperger's

The relevant research shows that the divorce rates for people with AS reaches a staggering 80%. The answer to the question why it is so high, may be found in how the symptoms of Asperger's affect intimate relationships. We have already discussed how people with AS find it difficult to understand others and express their feelings. They seem to lose interest in other people over time, they appear distant, their attitude is often mistaken to be self-centered and they are considered to be vain individuals.

These are not fair labels, as people with AS, due to their difficulties in understanding other people's emotional states, are usually shocked, upset and full of remorse when they are told that their actions were harmful or inappropriate!

Imagine the following scene to be the opening one of a movie: A woman enters a bedroom, walks around, opens a few drawers, and then leaves.

Most people could not watch this scene without wondering about the woman's behavior. Most people would think that maybe she was looking for something that should have been in the bedroom. Or maybe that she heard a noise and wanted to check it out. Or maybe, one could imagine, she had needed to go into the bathroom and forgot where she was going!

All these explanations are based on the suppositions about the woman's state of mind. In essence, an attempt was made to read her mind. Most people engage in such efforts all the time. Without these efforts, they would be "mind-blind," unaware that other people mentally exist, that thoughts themselves exist, and that others have emotions, intentions, memories and knowledge. They would be unable to make sense of the actions of another person.

Yet this is exactly what happens with the members of the social category called "aspies." Unfortunately, "mind-blindness" does not refer to science fiction. For people with AS, the term is all too real.

A successful romantic relationship can be difficult for anybody, either a normal person or an aspie. Consider all the books available that offer self-help in case of break-ups, the movies portraying cheating on a spouse and even one's own relationship history. After all the discussion in this book does anyone think that these difficulties would decrease for someone with Asperger's? Let's just say that, for these people, it's not the easiest of tasks to have a relationship while trying to function normally in the world.

Living with AS is harder upon aspies as they challenge their perfectionism and obsessive behavior. This does not preclude that it can also be a struggle for the people who are close to them. The symptoms associated with AS can be emotionally draining on both the aspie and his or her partner.

The absence of empathy may cause the other partner to feel isolated and lonely. A woman in love with a man with AS may read his difficulties to communicate and socialize as a lack of interest in the relationship. He may waver between gentleness and care all the way to coldness and distance. She may find his behavior difficult to understand, resulting in confusion and dissatisfaction.

Some common issues for people with a spouse or partner with AS include:

➢ A sense of segregation, because their relationship faces different challenges that are not easily understood by others

- After accepting that their partner's syndrome won't get better, they may feel guilt, disappointment and despair
- The previous stands true even if they accept that their partner won't recover from Asperger's
- Their own needs are not met in the relationship
- They may feel more responsible for their partner with AS than necessary
- Whether or not to end the relationship is a very frequent consideration
- Problems in the relationship don't improve despite many great efforts and this causes frustration
- Family members and friends don't fully understand or appreciate the extra strains placed on a relationship by Asperger's, so they do not offer their emotional and moral support

The best way to understand what it is to have a spouse with Asperger's is to read this story of a wife whose husband is an aspie:

"It has been hard to live with my husband, J. (the name is omitted for obvious reasons). He can be humorous at the same time as callus and

charming at the same time as self-centered and indifferent. When our children were small, I centered on them so his bad side did not trouble me. But now that they have left, he is truly driving me crazy!

We met when I was 17. He was handsome, sincere and brilliant-- and we fell in love rather quickly. We were quite different from each other, but I thought that my strengths balanced his weaknesses. I was organized and, I admit, just a little dominant. J. was the absent-minded type of a professor. He was studying for a degree in graphics, and would often work the entire night, forgetting to even eat or sleep. He became a lost puppy I wanted to save.

We had been dating for two years when I found out I was pregnant and we got married. After our children were born, I stayed home until they went to school, and then I got a part-time job at a nearby retail store. The children were always my top priority, and I focused virtually all of my energy on them.

J. and I have been having problems since the children were small. He did not know anything about parenting – not even how to take a temperature! He never could deal with any noise or disorder. If the children did not put their toys away, he would get angry. He would go crazy if any plans changed unexpectedly. Worst of all, he never really bonded with our children.

Once, when our daughter was in junior high school, she came home proud of a sketch of a boy's face she had drawn in art class. Instead of telling her how great it was, J. told her that the proportions of the face were all wrong, and used these words:

"Daughter, you have to learn the basics of physiology. The head is divided into five parts."

Who talks to a child that way?

Our daughter was in tears.

Every now and then, the original J. I fell deeply in love with reappeared, such as when our son was in a hospital for 3 months with a broken leg. He was 15 then, and J. was by his side every single day. He actually purchased the bicycle that our son wanted and took a photo of it. He gave the picture to our son to keep at the hospital as an "incentive to get well." At first I believed it was crazy – the child was in a cast! But I was wrong and it proved helpful.

Mainly, J. seems to live in his own world. I take care of everything from finances to maintenance as he cannot be trusted to complete anything. He cannot even keep his job. He is usually fighting with employers and co-workers. Not surprising, really. J. has never been able to handle people. If we go out with close friends, he will not even look at them. If anyone asks a question of him, he begins an endless rant. I am working two jobs now, but he seems completely unworried about how exhausted I am.

Just as I got at the point to break, an assistant gave me some articles regarding Asperger's that blew me away. Those who have it are quite intelligent – some of them are actually very talented – but have difficulty in conversation and bonding.

Due to the way their brain develops, they cannot understand interpersonal cues and often behave inappropriately or do not understand every day talk. The outline of it matched J. completely.

I'm not sure exactly where we go from here, though. If he does have the syndrome, it might explain his irritating habits. But will that make it any simpler to accept? You never know. J. and I have a long history. Deep down I realize we love each other. But unless something happens soon, I am going to go crazy!"

When it comes to making a choice whether the stay with a partner or a spouse with AS, it's time to consider the reasons that might make people want to stay together:

➢ Is change something too difficult to face?
➢ Is a divorce against someone's religion?
➢ For sake of the children?
➢ For reasons of safety and security?
➢ Would it cost too much or be too difficult to start over?
➢ Is there any fear of loneliness?
➢ Is there a concern of what others will think?

To begin with, the strategies required to be with a spouse or a partner with AS center around this aspect: the will to stay together. Everything else is a matter of training, teaching and learning.

From all the above examples it is obvious that while it may not be easy to deal with an aspie, with the proper teaching and learning process, they can be just as normal as everyone else.

Chapter 13: Adults with Asperger Syndrome

Asperger's Syndrome Diagnosis in Adults:

As mentioned earlier, Asperger's Syndrome is a condition that is not very easy to diagnose and the method of diagnoses depends on what age group you fall in and how much your situation has worsened.

One of the biggest issues with adults suffering from this syndrome is the fact that they believe in "self diagnosis," when they hear about or study this syndrome and try to draw parallels with their own conditions and symptoms and how they feel. Some often feel that they suffer from this condition just because a few symptoms match with their condition, and end up misdiagnosing the syndrome.

Sometimes it also happens that family members believe their loved ones, like an adult child, sibling, father, mother, spouse or spouse's sibling, may have Asperger's Syndrome but are not sure how to talk about this to them.

It should be remembered that Asperger's Syndrome, though difficult to understand, is not impossible to diagnose. Plus, self-diagnoses can have very harmful effects. The psychological factor comes into play here. If you do not suffer from this syndrome but you are of the idea that you do, you'll automatically begin to behave in a certain manner, and this may worsen your condition. This is why it is very important to get in touch with an expert and go through the proper channels to get this diagnosed.

What route should one go to if one fears the presence of AS? Many people do not know what to do and if pursuing an official diagnosis should be the first option. The answer is "yes." If you fear that you or anyone close to you have AS, you should not delay in going for an official check. Why? Let's discuss.

As mentioned earlier, one may go for a self-diagnosis with the help of materials available in books and on the internet. There are also several organizations like that of AANE that are out there to provide answers to questions related to the syndrome. However, the problem with such a diagnosis, as mentioned earlier, is the fact that you do not have the necessary skills and expertise to reach such a conclusion and a wrong conclusion can cause harm. Hence, professional help is needed. Also, seeking help should not be delayed because if you delay, you may have a difficult time due to the additional psychological issues as you'll spend a great amount of time thinking about and studying the situation and pressurizing your brain. Such an act may backfire and cause major issues.

There are several other reasons why it is important to diagnose this officially. These are:

> An official diagnosis is essential if one wishes to apply and avail themselves of Supplemental Security Income (SSI). The same goes for Social Security Disability Insurance (SSDI).

> An official diagnosis is essential if one wishes to apply for reasonable accommodation for employment under the Americans with Disabilities Act (ADA).

Now that the importance of an official diagnosis has been established, it is time to discuss how to get diagnosed. As mentioned earlier, a professional is needed, but there are several other points that should be taken care of. The answer to all your questions are given below:

One has the option to go to a psychiatrist (MD) or a neuropsychologist (PhD) to get tested. These experts generally prefer neuropsychological testing in order to build an opinion and reach a conclusion. This testing is fairly detailed and helps draw a picture about one's challenges and strengths to help in the diagnosis.

In addition to individuals with PhDs and/or MDs, others also have the ability to make a diagnosis. These include professionals that have the credentials to diagnose other related conditions. These include psychologists (MA), social workers (MSW) and other specialists that specialize in mental health.

Neuropsychological testing, even though important and helpful, is not mandatory for an "official diagnosis." Instead, one would need a written document, from the expert that diagnosed the condition, that clearly mentions that the individual suffers from AS. However, to be eligible for SSI, Asperger's Syndrome is not the only condition as those that suffer from other psychological issue may also apply for it without any psych testing.

Is it ever too late to seek diagnosis?

Better late than never is the saying which applies here. Getting diagnosed is all about being self-aware, and it is never too late to become self-aware. Once you are clear about your strengths and weaknesses, you will be in a position to use your strengths in a better fashion and to your own benefit. A diagnosis, no matter how late, will actually be beneficial as you will look at yourself and things from a different perspective and be able to overcome the odds. Understanding why you are the way you are will be of great help as having an explanation is better than having no answer.

However, if AS is diagnosed, it may impact a few things. For example, if your condition is diagnosed when you're ten, you will later be in a position to choose the right career in the light of your limitations. You can also plot your life in a better manner, choose the right degree, and study in a manner where you are not required to interact socially with a number of people.

The benefits of a diagnosis at a young age are understandably numerous. However, this does not mean that if it is diagnosed late, say when you're fifty, it is of no use. Even if it is late, you will be in a position to understand yourself and deal with others in a better manner. You can use the information to improve your relationships and do a life review. Plus, you can also change your environment and try to make new friends who are to your taste. Also, you can find others with similar conditions to share experiences and learn from each other. This is something that can be done online as well.

Also, even if you're older and you're diagnosed you can tell your family and friends about your condition and begin to see world a bit differently.

For Others:

If you think someone you know has this condition, waste no time and let someone know so they can get diagnosed. It is always better to know than to be unaware. The truth is that once you are aware of your condition, you will be able to improve it. If you're not aware, you will just live with it without doing anything to improve things.

If you do not know the reason why you are the way you are, you may blame it on other things, such as thinking that you're a failure or you're just not up to the mark. Whereas, when one has an explanation, things just fall into place and begin to make sense.

How to Tell?

This is a problem area as most people just do not know where to begin and they're afraid of looking rude or worsening things. The simple way is to focus on strengths and not weaknesses.

Firstly, be sure that you think the person has the syndrome. Of course, you cannot be sure unless they are diagnosed, but don't jump the gun and reach to conclusions right away. Conversely, once you're sure it is what you think it is, it's time to start the conversation.

> ➢ Start with the strengths. Go and talk to the person in a very normal manner, highlighting their strengths. For example, if you think your spouse has this issue you can go and highlight their positive qualities, like how they're able to remember dates and are very observant. This will motivate the individual and he or she will be interested in what you're about to say next.

> ➢ Now that you've started, it is time to move the topic to the weaknesses. It can go

something like "I really admire the way you never forget my birthday, but have you thought about your driving skills?" This is going from the positive to the negative in a subtle manner, without being rude. Here, you're not jumping to conclusions but opening an opportunity for discussion so that they're willing to converse and listen to you.

> Now it is time to tell them that you think they may have Asperger Syndrome without making this look critical. You will have to explain to them what this condition is and why you think they may have this condition. You may lead them to www.aane.org or other resources for further information. Provide support along the way.

> Once you tell them this, the reaction maybe negative or positive. Either the person will agree, thank you, and show interest in knowing more, or he or she will completely deny this and not believe a word you say. In both of these conditions, you should try to convince the person to

look into the fine details and pay a visit to a specialist for proper diagnosis.

➢ You should show the individual that you genuinely care so that they take your comments seriously and do something about it.

Contrary to the popular belief, individuals with Aspergers Syndrome can learn and improve their skills. The learning process may be slow and excruciating for some, but it is not impossible to teach them the art of communicating and handling themselves in public. The most important thing here is to have patience and few expectations. They will not behave the way you want them to within a few days. Unfortunately, they may never begin to behave the way you want them to, but there will surely be improvement and this is what counts.

The truth is that such individuals often have mixed feelings about improving their social skills. This may make them feel inferior or they may find it too difficult and unless they wish to improve, it is pointless to put in the effort.

This is because they often associate socializing with things like discouragement, failure, anxiety, depression, rejection and confusion. They may also have issues with people who are critical of them and not able to accept them for what they are. It may be difficult to convince them to learn social skills, but it may help if you can show them the benefits and somehow avoid reminders of these negative feelings.

This has to be done in a subtle manner, because when you tell them to learn they will feel as if you are looking down on them. They may ask why they have to learn or even why they have to be as good as others. These questions are provocative and complex, and though finding an answer may be difficult, you must answer these questions or you may not be able to move ahead.

These questions are provocative and complex, and though finding an answer may be difficult, you must answer these questions or you may not be able to move ahead.

They may also ask for a few things, such as friends that understand them and are willing to listen to them. At times, the demands may be too much but it is important to listen to them.

Make Peace with Traits

People that suffer from AS can live a normal life once they understand and come to term with this. There is no need to try to tell people you are something that you are not. Everybody wishes to get over their handicap or problem, but at the same time, it is important to accept what you are if you cannot do anything about it.

It is the responsibility of family and friends to stop making them feel any less than a human being and to treat them in a respectful manner without it seeming forced.

However, aspies should not use this as an excuse to stay the way they are because there's always an opportunity to change. Just because one has AS doesn't mean one can use it as an excuse to willfully avoid improvement. This label deserves some respect and power and should not merely be used as a tool to stay away from interactions with people.

Social Skills Explained

One of the biggest ways in which individuals with this syndrome suffer is social interaction. They fail to comprehend sentences and may come up with what are perceived as strange or rude remarks, which is also why they often fail to make friends. People may either find them boring or rude.

Such individuals need social situations broken down for proper understanding. They need to be explained a situation in detail and in simple words for them to be able to comprehend it. This may be repetitive, boring and also irritating, but this is what is required if you are dealing with such an individual.

These individuals will ask questions – a lot of questions – about people, things and also why people and things are the way they are. If they find something strange, they will not be able to adjust to it, and they'll require a rational explanation. This is very important because they will not feel comfortable unless they comprehend it.

So if an aspie is asked a question, he or she should ideally come up with a proper, rational response instead of just saying something like, "This is just the way I am." Such a statement may be technically true, but it appears standoffish and doesn't help to foster relationships.

This may get troublesome, as there are so many social rules, some of which even the general population doesn't always understand. Yet, the solution is to limit the sufferer's social interactions to an extent. There's no need for them to have dozens of friends. A few, good friends who understand their special needs should suffice.

Have a Mentor

As mentioned earlier, people with this syndrome ask a lot of questions, and some of us just do not have the nerve to handle all this. In such a situation, the right thing is to find them a mentor who will listen to them patiently and answer their questions, no matter how absurd. The person may be anyone from a professional to a friend or a family member.

All this will help the sufferer feel better as they will have someone to go to when they face any issues and they will also get answers to their questions. Plus, such a person may act as a therapist and give feedback on opinions and options to the sufferer. Also, this person will understand the sufferer better and can help others understand them as well.

Practice, Practice, and Practice

Practice is the key. Both you and the sufferer should practice and get to know each other better. If the sufferer is young, he or she should practice in the real world and try to mingle with the people at school.

If the person is an adult, he or she should try to mingle with the people at work and other such social gatherings, keeping the circle small. A large crowd may not be very pleasant.

Also, a few things may have to be explained to them and understood as well. Like, it isn't nice to outright ask people if they'd like to be friends. You must first talk to them to understand this. All this may be difficult for sufferers to understand but working with them you can help them learn the art.

Learn Social Skills

Those that suffer from this syndrome have issues learning social skills, but it doesn't mean they cannot learn these skills at all. The trial and error method also applies here.

Firstly, if you're communicating with someone with AS, you need to understand their limitations. Simply saying "share something about yourself" will not be enough because such a person will not be able to comprehend what this means or what it is you want them to share. Instead, you will have to ask them simple questions like, "What is your name?" and "What is your age?"

The trial and error method says that if you ask them a question and they fail to understand, explain it to them in a simple manner. They will ask you questions and they may even be able to learn something from you, but it is your duty not to give up but to explain to them what you're trying to ask.

Such people are used to certain responses and can only understand those types of interactions. For example, "How are you?" is a simple question that one may understand easily, but if you change it to something colloquial like, "How ya doing today, bro?" they may have difficulty in understanding what it means. Also, this changes from person to person, and some may find this too complex while others will not.

Instead of trying to explain things to aspies, you should change how you interact with them. Do not expect these individuals to begin to understand complex sentences. Instead, you should begin to use simple and specific sentences when interacting with them.

The rote approach is also helpful, which is why they may come up with the same responses. These people wish to make friends, but they fail to. If you understand how their brains work, you will easily be able to talk to them. Will this take time? Yes. How much? We don't know, but trying is the key here.

Also, this is not a rule of thumb. If you know someone with whom a different technique works, you should stick to it. Since people are different, the way they understand and interpret messages is different too.

Should You Tell Others About Asperger's?

One of the biggest challenges that aspies and their families have is if they should tell others about their condition or not. There's no one definite answer to this question because there are both pros and cons.

Firstly, the biggest advantage is that if one is aware of your condition, they will be more thoughtful towards you and understand your limitations, and hence have more reasonable expectations regarding interactions. Also, they will know how to deal with you and may help you acquire social and other skills.

However, as mentioned earlier, there is a negative side as well. Unfortunately, not everyone will understand the situation, and some may get critical or start to make fun of the situation. To tell or not to tell depends on a number of things, especially with whom you are talking to and how comfortable you are with the revelation. Many people refrain from disclosing their condition mostly due to how they fear they might be treated, even though in some situations it has been proven to be beneficial. Also, the more people know about the condition the more awareness there will be in society as a whole. Conversely, not telling ANYONE about the situation at all and keeping it to yourself is a big mistake. There should be people that know what you suffer from and go through as you will need such people to support you in life.

The biggest issue here is the one of expectation. If one is not aware of the condition and limitations, he or she will automatically have high expectations from the aspie, and if those expectations are not met, there will be issues. In such a situation, it will be wise to speak about it.

Asperger Syndrome and Sexual Codes of Conduct

As mentioned in cases explained earlier, those that suffer from Asperger's Syndrome may have issues understanding sex, and they may have many questions related to it. Unfortunately, however, this topic is new and research on this is in its initial stage.

Contrary to the popular belief, individuals with Asperger's Syndrome have an interest in sex, but the main issue arises in understanding and comprehending it. Many believe that they get confused due to a number of skills one needs in order to have an intimate relationship.

Because individuals with Asperger's syndrome have poor comprehension skills, they may often have an incorrect, immature, delayed or inappropriate understanding of the sexual codes of conduct. They may fail to understand what acceptable sexually behavior is and where the boundaries lie. The failure to understand the sexual code of conduct may often cause sexually inappropriate behavior. For example, an individual that suffers from this syndrome may not understand that it is not socially acceptable to display "sexual behavior" in public.

Individuals that have AS but are living a good life with successful careers may have trouble understanding relationships and sex due to the complexities attached.

The Workplace and Asperger's Syndrome

As mentioned in the cases, those that suffer from AS syndrome can work and live a normal life if they have the right support system. However, the number of workplace opportunities available to them is limited. Nonetheless, there are several job opportunities they can avail and use their skills and capabilities in the best possible manner.

What is important is to realize what they are good at and then try their hands at it. Understandably, there are a few options that may be completely out of the person's abilities. Hence, one should look at options that are possible and can be attained. Instead of thinking, "I cannot work," their attitude should be to look for jobs they can do well in, and then prepare for them. To help you pick the right career path, below are some suggestions:

Career Options for Visual Thinkers

The below mentioned career options may sound difficult but are easily attainable. Since those that suffer from Asperger's Syndrome have excellent memory, the craft can be learnt easily.

- ➢ Computer programming
- ➢ Photography
- ➢ Drafting
- ➢ Commercial art
- ➢ Equipment design
- ➢ Appliance repair
- ➢ Mechanic
- ➢ Handcraft artisan
- ➢ Video game designer
- ➢ Webpage designer
- ➢ Building trades
- ➢ Building maintenance

If one is good at math or music, he or she can try a different route. Some options that such patients have include:

- Accounting
- Engineering
- Computer programming
- Journalist, copy editor
- Musical instrument tuner
- Taxi driver
- Statistician
- Filing positions
- Bank teller
- Mathematician
- Telemarketing

Conclusion

We have tried to give as comprehensive of a presentation of Asperger Syndrome as possible. This is a condition where neither the causes have been uncovered, nor has a definite cure has been devised by science and research. This is a disorder in which patients may be withdrawn, aggressive, impulsive, with restrictive and repetitive behavior patterns, linguistic and comprehension inadequacies and cognitive dysfunctions.

But it's also a condition that could lead to great things; one that can even help patients display significant skills and acquire potential for great accomplishments in life, perhaps even winning a Nobel Prize. This is a condition that counts many notable authors, esteemed mathematicians and distinguished theoretical physicists in its ranks.

Should we call Asperger's a disorder? Or should we comply with the wishes of the people that exhibit its symptoms and call them different? Should we put them under the same classification as homosexuals, as they ask? Or should we consider them as people that need assistance and healing, as their parents think when they are children and they are diagnosed with the syndrome?

Throughout the book we respected the term they chose for themselves, aspies, and we have used it in our presentation. We have also mentioned the legal implications that exist should they be considered merely "different," as well as Simon Baron-Cohen's opinion that there are two very compelling reasons that their categorization as patients should remain.

For those who put the right of self-disposition above all else, they should be considered as different. For those who oppose the existence of an "ideal" human standard (probably because of the influence of what happened the last time someone considered certain anthropological characteristics as superior and others as inferior), like an "ideal" configuration of the brain, they should also be considered different.

Self-disposition requires a level of self-awareness and the ability to defend oneself, to be able to distinguish what is right and what is wrong. In a great number of the people that display AS, the case is that they either have no self-awareness at all, or very little of it, and they cannot defend themselves, making them good prospects for victimization, manipulation and bullying. As for the distinction between right and wrong, they have their own criteria, which may vary greatly from what the rest of the world and society in general consider as such.

So it's actually a question of practicality. If they can take care of themselves and present no danger to themselves and to others as the law requires, then their wishes should be respected and they should be reclassified from "patients" to "different." But if none of the above is true or valid, they should be considered as patients in need of medical assistance and supervision.

Neither traditional nor alternative medicine deals with the core problem. If they did, there would be no debate. All that the existing therapies do is address and reduce the symptoms and their common bases: the human brain and its complex functions, neuron connections and input translation centers.

Perhaps the Chinese view of the body and mind as a single undivided entity is a better consideration. Or it could be possible that the way Ayurveda is treating the syndrome is based on a better foundation than Western medicine. Or, the case could be that parts of the truth exist in each different view and by putting these parts together, the different views and philosophies may provide an answer.

In the end, it all comes down to simplicity. ***Whatever works is good enough!*** It does not matter where it comes from. If the condition is rectified and the aspie can take care of his or her own needs after being subjected to a certain set of treatments, this philosophy is good enough for this specific individual. Another set of therapies may work for another aspie. It will also be good enough for him or her as well.

The final piece of advice that we can offer our readers is that no matter what the choice of treatment might be, it will need three elements for it to work:

A) **PATIENCE**
B) **PERSISTENCE**
C) **TIME**

When there is self-awareness and knowledge of the ailment which troubles the individual, the most imperative aspect of any therapy is that ***the patient cannot go through it without***

BELIEVING that it will be effective. Going through any therapy under the notion that nothing works and that everything is in vain follows logically that everything will not work and that the therapy will not be effective. However, it's not because it's a bad or an incorrect therapy. It will be so because the patient themselves want it to be so.

In the case of Asperger's (and all forms of autism for that matter), the same holds true for those who are supposed to offer support and assistance, like parents, siblings and teachers. Because aspies may not be self-aware, or have an informed knowledge about their condition, it is their families and friends who must learn to be patient and persistent. It is their loved ones who must communicate the message to the individual with AS. If they are impatient and give up too easily, so will the aspie. That negates the point of the exercise.

Thank you again for reading this book!

I hope this book was able to help you.

Thank you and good luck!

Bibliography

1. Akshoomoff N, Pierce K, Courchesne E. The neurobiological basis of autism from a developmental perspective. Development and Psychopathology, 2002; 14: 613-634.

2. American Academy of Pediatrics Committee on Children With Disabilities. The pediatrician's role in the diagnosis and management of autistic spectrum disorder in children. Pediatrics, 2001; 107(5): 1221-1226.

3. American Psychiatric Association. Diagnostic and statistical manual of mental disorders: DSM-IV-TR (fourth edition, text revision). Washington DC: American Psychiatric Association, 2000.

4. Autism Society of America. Biomedical and Dietary Treatments (Fact Sheet) [cited 2004], 2003. Bethesda, MD: Autism Society of America. Available from: http://www.autism-society.org/site/PageServer?pagename=Biomedi calDietaryTreatments.

5. Baird G, Charman T, Baron-Cohen S, Cox A, Swettenham J, Wheelwright S, Drew A. A screening instrument for autism at 18 months of

age: A 6-year follow-up study. Journal of the American Academy of Child and Adolescent Psychiatry, 2000; 39: 694-702.

6. Berument SK, Rutter M, Lord C, Pickles A, Bailey A. Autism Screening Questionnaire: diagnostic validity. British Journal of Psychiatry, 1999; 175: 444-451.

7. Couper JJ, Sampson AJ. Children with autism deserve evidence-based intervention. Medical Journal of Australia, 2003; 178: 424-425.

8. Courchesne E. Carper R, Akshoomoff N. Evidence of brain overgrowth in the first year of life in autism. JAMA, 2003; 290(3): 337-344.

9. Department of Health and Human Services. Mental Health: A Report of the Surgeon General. Rockville, MD: Department of Health and Human Services, Substance Abuse and Mental Health Services Administration, Center for Mental Health Services, National Institute of Mental Health, 1999.

10. Dunlap G, Foxe L. Teaching students with autism. ERIC EC Digest #E582, 1999 October.

11. Ehlers S, Gillberg C, Wing L. A screening questionnaire for Asperger syndrome and other

high-functioning autism spectrum disorders in school age children. Journal of Autism and Developmental Disorders, 1999; 29(2): 129-141.

12. Families and Fragile X Syndrome: U.S. Department of Health and Human Services, Public Health Service, National Institutes of Health, National Institute of Child Health and Human Development. 2003

13. Filipek PA, Accardo PJ, Ashwal S, Baranek GT, Cook Jr. EH, Dawson G, Gordon B, Gravel JS, Johnson CP, Kallen RJ, Levy SE, Minshew NJ, Ozonoff S, Prizant BM, Rapin I, Rogers SJ, Stone WL, Teplin SW, Tuchman RF, Volkmar FR. Practice parameter: screening and diagnosis of autism. Neurology, 2000; 55: 468-479.

14. Filipek PA, Accardo PJ, Baranek GT, Cook Jr. EH, Dawson G, Gordon B, Gravel JS, Johnson CP, Kellen RJ, Levy SE, Minshew NJ, Prizant BM, Rapin I, Rogers SJ, Stone WL, Teplin S, Tuchman RF, Volkmar FR. The screening and diagnosis of autism spectrum disorders. Journal of Autism and Developmental Disorders, 1999; 29(2): 439-484.

15. Garnett MS, Attwood AJ. The Australian scale for Asperger's syndrome. In: Attwood,

Tony. Asperger's Syndrome: A Guide for Parents and Professionals. London: Jessica Kingsley Publishers, 1997.

16. Korvatska E, Van de Water J, Anders TF, Gershwin ME. Genetic and immunologic considerations in autism. Neurobiology of Disease, 2002; 9: 107-125.

17. Lord C, Risi S, Lambrecht L, Cook EH, Leventhal BL, DiLavore PC, Pickles A, Rutter M. The autism diagnostic observation schedule-generic: a standard measure of social and communication deficits associated with the spectrum of autism. Journal of Autism and Developmental Disorders, 2000; 30(3): 205-230.

18. Lovaas OI. Behavioral treatment and normal educational and intellectual functioning in young autistic children. Journal of Consulting and Clinical Psychology, 1987; 55: 3-9.

19. McDougle CJ, Stigler KA, Posey DJ. Treatment of aggression in children and adolescents with autism and conduct disorder. Journal of Clinical Psychiatry, 2003; 64 (supplement 4): 16-25.

20. McEachin JJ, Smith T, Lovaas OI. Long-term outcome for children with autism who received early intensive behavioral treatment. American Journal on Mental Retardation, 1993; 97: 359-372.

21. Newschaffer CJ (Johns Hopkins Bloomberg School of Public Health). Autism Among Us: Rising Concerns and the Public Health Response [Video on the Internet]. Public Health Training Network, 2003 June 20. Available from: http://www.publichealthgrandrounds.unc.edu/autism/webcast.htm.

22. Powers MD. What Is Autism? In: Powers MD, ed. Children with Autism: A Parent's Guide, Second Edition. Bethesda, MD: Woodbine House, 2000, 28.

23. Research Units on Pediatric Psychopharmacology Network. Risperidone in children with autism and serious behavioral problems. New England Journal of Medicine, 2002; 347(5): 314-321.

24. Robbins DI, Fein D, Barton MI, Green JA. The modified checklist for autism in toddlers: an initial study investigating the early detection of autism and pervasive developmental disorders.

Journal of Autism and Developmental Disorders, 2001; 31(2): 149-151.

25. Scott FJ, Baron-Cohen S, Bolton P, Brayne C. The Cast (Childhood Asperger Syndrome Test): preliminary development of a UK screen for mainstream primary-school-age children. Autism, 2002; 2(1): 9-31.

26. Smalley SI, Autism and tuberous sclerosis. Journal of Autism and Developmental Disorders, 1998; 28(5): 407-414.

27. Stone WL, Coonrod EE, Ousley OY. Brief report: screening tool for autism in two-year-olds (STAT): development and preliminary data. Journal of Autism and Developmental Disorders, 2000; 30(6): 607-612.

28. Tadevosyan-Leyfer O, Dowd M, Mankoski R, Winklosky B, Putnam S, McGrath L, Tager-Flusberg H, Folstein SE. A principal components analysis of the autism diagnostic interview-revised. Journal of the American Academy of Child and Adolescent Psychiatry, 2003; 42(7): 864-872.

29. Van Bourgondien ME, Marcus LM, Schopler E. Comparison of DSM-III-R and childhood autism rating scale diagnoses of autism. Journal

of Autism and Developmental Disorders, 1992; 22(4): 493-506.

30. Volkmar FR. Medical Problems, Treatments, and Professionals. In: Powers MD, ed. Children with Autism: A Parent's Guide, Second Edition. Bethesda, MD: Woodbine House, 2000; 73-74.

31. Yeargin-Allsopp M, Rice C, Karapurkar T, Doernberg N, Boyle C, Murphy C. Prevalence of Autism in a US Metropolitan Area. The Journal of the American Medical Association.. 2003 Jan 1;289(1):49-55.

55677593R00128

Made in the USA
Middletown, DE
18 July 2019